A New Body in
4 Weeks

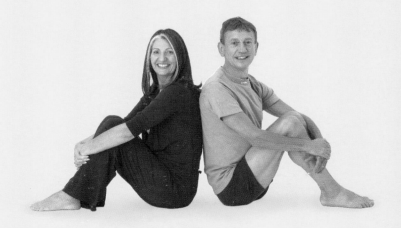

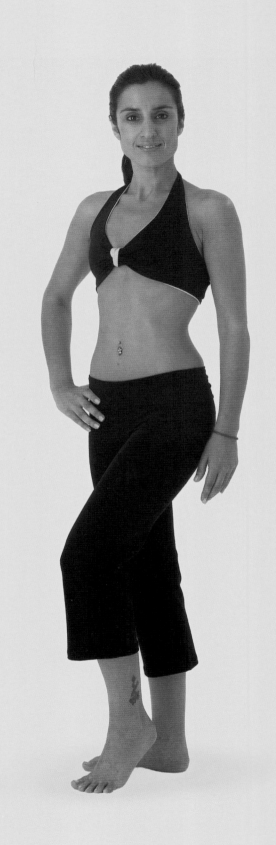

A New Body in
4 Weeks

Get the figure you've always
wanted with the all-new
Body Control Pilates® Programme

Lynne
Robinson

Gordon
Thomson

PAN BOOKS

First published 2005 by Pan Books
an imprint of Pan Macmillan Ltd
Pan Macmillan, 20 New Wharf Road, London N1 9RR
Basingstoke and Oxford
Associated companies throughout the world
www.panmacmillan.com

ISBN 0 330 43512 4

Photography by Paul Bricknell
Illustrations by Atomic Squib Ltd
Technical illustrations by Raymond Turvey

A CIP catalogue record for this book is available from
the British Library.

Designed by Rafaela Romaya
Printed and bound in Great Britain by Bath Press

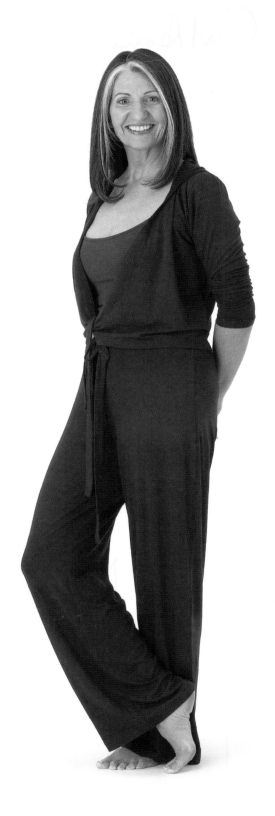

Contents

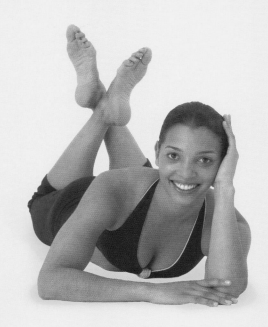

Acknowledgements

When Gordon and I wrote our first book, *Body Control the Pilates Way*, we passionately believed in the power of Pilates, but neither of us could have guessed just how successful the book would be or how popular Pilates would become. Seventeen books later, you would think we would have run out of ideas! Yet, as long-suffering Jacqui, Rafi and Liz from Pan Macmillan will testify, we have had to cut down the original manuscript for this book leaving out many favourite exercises. Where do we get our inspiration? Quite simply, from our clients and our teachers.

The beauty of the Body Control approach to Pilates is in the way it breaks down the classical, complex, choreographed exercises into simple tasks. These simple tasks educate the client in good movement skills. As we work with clients, we find ourselves discovering new and exciting ways to teach the exercises. Every 'body' is different and a good teacher is challenged constantly to find new ways to build strength and flexibility and to make their classes stimulating. Many of the exercises in this book have been created in answer to our clients' needs.

We have trained about 600 Body Control Pilates teachers worldwide, and I am immensely proud of each and every one of them. All our teachers undergo extensive training to earn the right to use the term Body Control Pilates in connection with their teaching, yet they are all, without exception, dedicated to furthering their knowledge and teaching expertise. Every professional development workshop or course we run is oversubscribed, a sign that our teachers remain hungry for knowledge! Some of the new variations and combinations of exercises in this pro-gramme were inspired by our teachers. In particular, I would like to take this opportunity to thank Lisa Bradshaw, Sarah Marks and Catherine Wilks for their immense contri-butions to Body Control Pilates.

Pilates changed the shape of my body and the direction of my life. I am thrilled that others can now enjoy Pilates through this book, our other books and DVDs and also through our teachers.

Gordon and I would like to thank the stunning models who kindly agreed to appear in this book: Yasmeen, Zoe, Emma Jane and Simone, you look gorgeous!

Lynne Robinson

Since my mum's passing away two years ago, I would like to dedicate my share in this work to my father.

My thanks go to the editorial team at Macmillan (Rafi Romaya and Jacqui Butler) who have again crafted a wonderfully elegant book. We hope this can help bring Pilates to an ever-increasing audience and make a new group of people aware of such an important technique for the twenty-first century.

It is eight years since Lynne and I wrote our first book *Body Control The Pilates Way* and thirty years ago that I was first introduced to the technique by Alan Herdman in his studio at London Contemporary Dance.

I have been directing and teaching in my own studio in South Kensington for twenty years now and this experience still gives me personal support and a sense of fulfilment which I cannot imagine doing without – thank you to clients old and new and especially to my staff Cheryl, Ellie, Judy, Patricia, Richard, Laurence, Simone, Sue, Linda, Lisa, Amanda, Jenny and Sam who make it work like magic.

Body Control Pilates has been a resounding success, based above all on the talent and hard work of the teacher training staff and students, and indeed everyone behind the scenes who has created a uniquely accessible product. In particular, I must express my gratitude to and admiration for Lynne and Leigh who have worked endless gruelling hours to build up the company over this last decade.

Gordon Thomson

A New Body in 4 Weeks

By selecting this book we're assuming you would like a new body in four weeks.

Perhaps you aren't happy with your figure, or there is something about your body you would like to change. Perhaps you are going on holiday and the bikini threatens. Or maybe you have a special event coming up which requires you to look your best.

Can it be done? The answer is yes! And before you consider cosmetic surgery, we would like a chance to change your body naturally, using the Body Control Pilates method of exercise.

All we need is four weeks of your time and a commitment to practise for 45 minutes five times a week. Far less painful than recovering from surgery and considerably easier on your bank balance! What's more, you might even enjoy it! Of course, you may not want such a tight deadline – in which case you can spread the programme over an eight- or even a twelve-week period. The key to success lies in doing an absolute minimum of 3 x 45 minute workouts a week, but ideally 5 x 45 minutes.

'In ten sessions you will feel a difference, in twenty you will see the difference and in thirty you will have a whole new body.' Joseph Pilates

If you have ever wondered why you see so much about Pilates in the press, why there are now so many Pilates books and videos and why so many people are talking about Pilates, the answer is simple: it works! Pilates has had A-list celebrity fans for over ninety years. People like Lauren Bacall and the late Katharine Hepburn were early advocates of the method and many celebrities still follow this unique regime, seduced by the fabulous, long, lean look that can be achieved.

But how much can a body change in just four weeks and how will your body continue to change in the months that follow? Well, the first four weeks of this programme are, in fact, the most important because it is during this time that you will lay down the foundations of your new body.

After your very first session your body will wake up. You will notice that you are more body-aware. In particular, you will be aware of your posture. Never underestimate just how awful bad posture looks: it is so unflattering. Think about it. When you stand in front of a mirror what do you do? You automatically stand upright and pull your stomach in because it makes you look taller and slimmer and your clothes look better when your shoulders are open and back. But then what do you do when you walk away from the mirror? Do you carry on walking tall and pulling your stomach in? Only if you think someone is watching you! We all have two kinds of posture, one for an audience and our usual one.

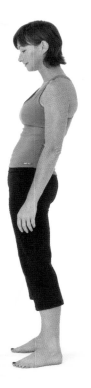

Bad Posture

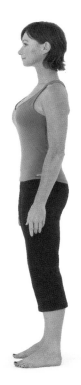

Good Posture

What Pilates can do is to change your posture fundamentally so you stand and move with grace and elegance all the time, not just for an audience. The effect is dramatic. However, standing properly and pulling your stomach in takes a lot of effort. You couldn't keep it up all day, or could you? This is where Pilates can help, it not only teaches you how to be aware of good posture, it also gives your muscles the strength to maintain that posture all day.

Some of the muscles you use to maintain good posture are your deep abdominals, and these are the same muscles which hold the key to having a flat stomach. Pilates is famous for giving you a longer, leaner torso because in the course of one session you do literally hundreds of abdominal exercises as you learn to keep your deep abdominals engaged while you do all the exercises. It means you will be creating your very own natural corset that wraps around your middle and holds you in: a built-in girdle of strength.

It is from this strong centre that you will learn to make slow, controlled movements. These movements are deceiving. They look simple and yet they are remarkably effective at toning problem areas such as the buttocks, inner and outer thighs and the upper arms. The reason they are so effective is that you build your strength from the inside out, focusing first on good alignment and then on the deep stabilizing muscles which create a foundation on which to tone the more superficial muscles. By taking time to ensure you use your muscles correctly, you work with the body's natural movement patterns, restoring the balance lost by poor posture, misuse or lack of use. The slow pace of the exercises actually makes them

harder to do. After just a few sessions you will notice that you are firming up all over.

Not only will your body be more stream-lined, it will also be more supple and stronger.

The list of benefits is almost endless:

- a firmer, flatter stomach
- improved posture
- greater flexibility
- toned arms and shoulders
- a defined waist
- firmer buttocks and thighs
- less cellulite
- more efficient breathing
- stronger back muscles
- better alignment
- better core strength
- improved balance
- better co-ordination
- greater bone density
- mobile joints
- improved circulation
- more energy
- stress relief
- an enhanced sex life
- a sense of well-being

Over the next few weeks you can expect dramatic changes to your body shape. One of the main differences between this book and our previous books is that we will be helping you determine which exercises are right for your particular shape. In this way you can personalize your workouts, choosing exercises which target your problem areas. For example, there may be parts of your body which are too slim and need to be developed. If your hips are very narrow, you might want to define your waist and streamline your upper body so your hips look more rounded. You may even want to sculpt your bottom so it looks more rounded. You might actually think your body is too muscular and needs a 'softer' look, but still want it to be toned. This book will enable you to design your own body, working with what nature has already given you.

In order to help you achieve this change in shape in a few weeks we have created some exciting new exercises and designed new variations on existing favourites. They have been chosen specifically for their effectiveness in toning the body. The focus in this book, unlike in some of our previous books, is to get the best cosmetic results in the shortest possible time.

It is not without reason that celebrities turn to Pilates when they have a nude scene coming up in a new movie. It avoids the embarrassment of needing a body double!

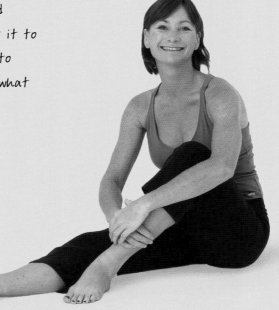

How to Use this Book

1
STEP

After you have decided which body shape you are (page 9) read through the advice given for your shape: pear (page 10), apple (page 11), rectangular (page 12) and pencil (page 13).

2
STEP

Work out and make a note of your BMI (page 23). Check this again after a few weeks, it will indicate how your body is changing.

3
STEP

Read through the General Guidelines for Aerobic Exercise (page 24).

4
STEP

Read through the Eight Principles of Body Control Pilates (page 27); it will give you a better understanding of why you are working in such a precise way. Then read through the Basics of Body Control Pilates chapter (page 33) and practise the exercises until you are confident you have mastered the basic skills.

Even if you are already familiar with Pilates it makes good sense to revise these basic skills regularly; even the most devoted Pilates disciple (teachers included) benefits from revisiting the basic exercises from time to time.

5
STEP

Once you have practised and mastered the basic exercises you are ready to start the programme designed for your body shape. Your four weeks start from this point. The exercises are described on pages 65–121, grouped according to which body parts they target most.

For each body shape there is a four-week schedule of balanced workouts. You must do 5 x 45 minute workouts a week adding up to a total of 3 hours 45 minutes. Each 45-minute workout is perfectly balanced, but will also target the particular problem areas of your body shape. To this you must add cardiovascular sessions of 2 or 3 x 30 continuous minutes twice a week and 3 x 10 minutes sessions on the other days.

Your workouts for each week change subtly so you will continue to tone and sculpt the whole body while at the same time progressing your Pilates skills.

During these four weeks you will lay the foundations of your new body – take your time to learn the exercises thoroughly. If you hurry an exercise or workout you will be wasting your time. Our exercises only work when you do them in a controlled way!

We have also given you a few advanced exercises. It is our hope that you will enjoy this programme so much that you will wish to continue Pilates beyond the four-week period. With this in mind, we have added just a few exercises which require excellent core stability, flexibility and co-ordination.

Joseph Pilates and the Origins of the Pilates Method

The Pilates Method was developed by the late Joseph Hubertus Pilates. Born in Germany in 1880, he was so sickly as a child, suffering from rickets, asthma and rheumatic fever, that his doctors predicted he would not survive his fifth birthday. But instead of wrapping him in cotton wool, his enlightened parents encouraged him to play outdoors. His health improved dramatically and, perhaps as a consequence, he became obsessed with physical fitness to improve his body image. He was a keen sportsman, and many elements from his wide range of interests, including martial arts, yoga and gymnastics, found their way into his fitness programme. His main source of income was teaching self-defence. It was while he was teaching the police at Scotland Yard that the First World War broke out. Because of his nationality, he was interned for the duration of the war. Many of the remedial exercises stem from this time when he taught fitness to his fellow internees.

Returning to Germany after the war, he started to become involved in, and introduced his exercises to, the world of dance. In 1926 Joseph moved to the USA to distance himself from the unfolding events in his home country, and proceeded to set up his first fitness studio in New York at an address he shared with the New York City Ballet.

His original clients were boxers, but it wasn't long before he was working with leading ballet dancers, because his exercises were felt to perfect and complement their traditional exercise programme. He must have looked a strange figure, often teaching in his swimming trunks and not afraid to give very robust correction to clients during their sessions. His ideas and approach have been shown to be years ahead of his time because, today, the Pilates Method is a core part of the training programme for a wide range of elite athletes and performers, and is also supported by medical specialists.

Joseph Pilates died in 1967, his death being caused indirectly by the effects of a fire at his studio. His legacy was to leave a method of body conditioning that was never precisely laid down, but which has been developed and expanded by the teachers who have come after him.

I am a sculptor who specializes in producing large-scale installations for film and TV sets. That makes for a mix of physical and mental challenges – I have to manoeuvre heavy objects in all weathers and at all times of the day and night, while still maintaining my concentration and creativity.

I first came to Gordon more than twenty years ago with a severe lower-back problem which was threatening to incapacitate me, and I have regularly sought his help since then.

Pilates has strengthened my body and enabled me to use it without fear. I believe that this method can be an enormous bonus to anyone who is under pressure or who simply wants to live life to the maximum.

Lolly Batty, Sculptor

The Development of Body Control Pilates

The Body Control Pilates method is closely based on the work of Joseph Pilates, but is unique in the way it prepares the body for what are known as the classical Pilates exercises, many of which are far too advanced for the average person new to Pilates.

Our approach is based on the belief that the necessary skills and movements should be taught progressively, building layer upon layer, towards the end result of performing the intermediate and advanced exercises safely and effectively. We have also broken the exercises down so they can be done by an average body, rather than only by people who come from the worlds of dance or sport, the traditional disciplines of Pilates enthusiasts. It is this approach that has won the support of many of the leading medical bodies and of several athletes and governing bodies in sport.

Body Control Pilates was founded and registered as a trademark in 1996 by Lynne Robinson and Gordon Thomson, ahead of the publication in March 1997 of Lynne and Gordon's first book *Body Control the Pilates Way* (a book of which there were only humble expectations, yet which quickly became an international exercise bestseller). We subsequently established our first training course for people wanting to learn to teach the Body Control Pilates method.

Ten years on, it is hard to remember just what pioneering days those were, because today Pilates is one of the most popular of exercise regimes. Barely a week goes by without a celebrity mention in the national media. Body Control Pilates is now the in-flight exercise pro-gramme for British Airways; it is promotionally linked with major consumer brands such as Kellogg's; and used by the GB rowing team including the Olympic gold medal rowers. You can probably find a qualified teacher close to you, because the Body Control Pilates Association has more than 700 members, all of whom have undergone extensive training to gain certification in teaching the Body Control Pilates method. To retain this certification, Body Control Pilates teachers also have to undertake further professional development studies every year.

As the geographical reach of Body Control Pilates has grown as a result of international book-publishing deals and Lynne's videos, so we have started to build teaching and support activities in parts of the world as varied as North America, Australia, South Africa, Spain, Portugal and Poland.

Underpinning this rapid expansion, our prime focus has continued to be on the development of teaching skills and knowledge – ensuring everyone working within the Body Control Pilates 'family' has access to the latest knowledge with regard to relevant research and techniques – and, last but not least, that the numerous benefits of Pilates remain accessible to as wide a segment of the population as possible, through our network of teachers and through our books and videos.

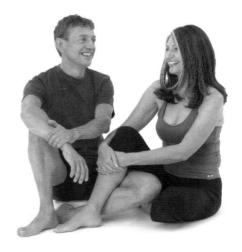

Before You Begin

- Be sure you have no pressing unfinished business.
- Take the telephone off the hook or put the answering machine on.
- You may prefer silence, otherwise put on some unobtrusive classical or new-age music.
- Wear something warm and comfortable, allowing free movement.
- Barefoot is best, non-slip socks otherwise.
- The best time to exercise is usually in the late afternoon or evening when your muscles are already warmed up as a result of the day's activity. Exercising in the morning is fine, but you will need to take longer to warm up thoroughly. Be flexible, as you will probably need to adjust the timing according to how you feel.

Please do not exercise if you:
- are feeling unwell or tired
- have just eaten a heavy meal
- have been drinking alcohol
- are in pain
- are feeling nauseous

You will need:
- hand-held weights of 0.5–4 kg (1–10 lb approx.) each and leg weights of 0.5–1 kg (1– 2.5 lb approx.) each
- a padded non-slip mat
- space to work in
- a folded towel or a small flat pillow
- a plump pillow
- a tennis ball
- a scarf, long towel or stretch band
- loose, comfortable clothing and bare feet
- a sturdy chair

It is always wise to consult your doctor before taking up a new exercise regime. You should be aware that not all the exercises are suitable for use during pregnancy. If you have a back problem you will need to consult your medical practitioner. Many of the exercises are wonderful for back-related problems, but you should always take expert advice.

It is our hope that you will use this book and the workouts for a lot longer than four weeks. With this in mind, we have given you a few advanced exercises. Rowing, Curled-Up Leg Beats and Stretching Mermaid 2 are all exercises that require excellent core stability and flexibility. It may take you months (or even years!) to reach this level.

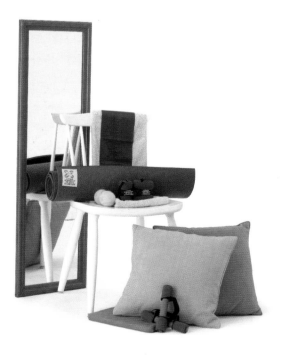

Determining Your Body Shape

Before you start, you need to take an honest look at your body and decide what you want to change. You need to be realistic. Your body shape, height, weight, strength, flexibility, even your co-ordination and movement skills are all influenced by a variety of things ranging from inherited factors, your health and diet, to your work, hobbies and habits. The chances are that you have inherited more than your hair colour from your parents; if your mother was short and pear-shaped there is a strong chance you are too. You may also have a similar posture and her way of moving because you copied her when you were young. This does not mean, however, that you are stuck with being short, pear-shaped and round shouldered for ever – by choosing this book you have taken the first step to changing these things and making the best of what nature has handed you.

When determining which exercise is going to suit you, it is invaluable to know what you can and can't change. For example, large bones are large bones, and no amount of exercise will reduce them. However, with an understanding of your body shape you can adjust your workouts to get maximum results.

To decide which body shape you are and to determine what are your good and bad areas you will need mirrors. Most of us are very familiar with what we look like from the front and the side, but few of us pay much attention to the back view and it may come as a bit of a shock! If you can, set up some mirrors at home so you can see yourself from every angle. If this isn't possible, you could try using the changing rooms in a clothes shop – they often have two or three mirrors positioned so you can get an all-round view. You will need to strip down to your underwear to get the true image. Compare what you see against the different body shapes to find out which one is nearest your shape. Take note of any areas of your body that really need extra attention.

The different shapes we have given you to choose from are:

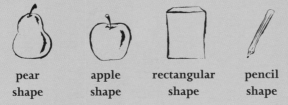

| pear shape | apple shape | rectangular shape | pencil shape |

Let's look at each shape in more detail, noting not just what you see in the mirror but also other factors such as how flexible you are and how easy it is for you to lose weight.

The Pear Shape

This is the most common female shape and is easily recognizable. You will probably love buying tops, but hate it when you have to buy trousers!

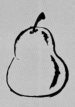

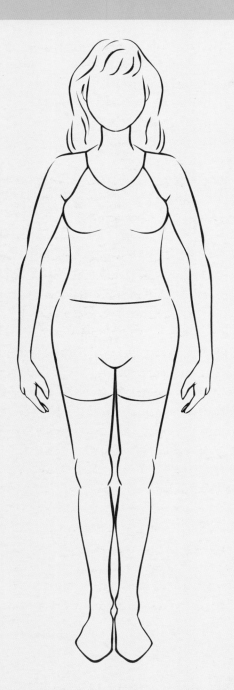

- You tend to carry weight on your hips, thighs, abdomen and the backs of your arms.
- You eat little, but you store it all.
- Your metabolism is slow.
- You have trouble losing weight.
- You have large bones.
- You have good muscle endurance.
- Your cardiovascular system is good.
- You have a medium heart rate.

Now, the good news is that you have a lot of natural strength in your body especially in your lower half. We can use this to your advantage.

The Apple Shape

As you can see, many of your characteristics are similar to the pear shape, with the obvious exception that you also store fat around your waist, which is more likely to be linked with health problems than fat stored on your hips.

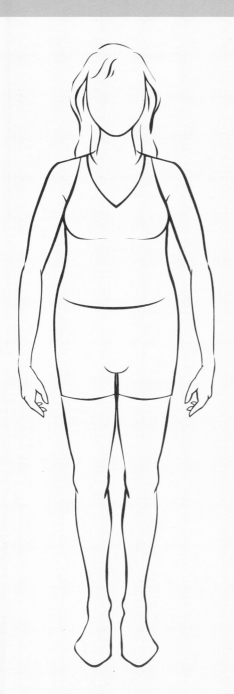

- You tend to carry weight around your middle as well as on your hips, thighs, abdomen and the backs of your arms.
- You eat little, but you store it all.
- Your metabolism is slow.
- You have trouble losing weight.
- You have large bones.
- You have good muscle endurance.
- Your cardiovascular system is good.
- You have a medium heart rate.

Fat stored round the waist can give rise to an increased risk of non-insulin diabetes, heart disease, high blood pressure and abnormal blood-fat levels. In women, central obesity is also associated with a higher risk of pre-menopausal breast cancer. The reason why the apple-shaped distribution of fat is more harmful to health than the pear-shaped distribution is not clearly understood. One theory is that central fat is more metabolically active, causing changes in the levels of blood fats, which increase the risk of heart disease. However, certain factors such as smoking and drinking alcohol seem to increase the likelihood of fat being laid down in the stomach area, while exercise helps reduce stomach fat.

Clearly, our focus when designing your programme will be all-over body conditioning with a special focus on your midriff area.

Body Shapes

The Rectangular Shape

From an athletic point of view, your body shape and type is ideal.
You can build muscle quickly and burn fat easily, making you
a natural sportswoman. You are better at sprinting than long-distance
running because you find endurance sports challenging.

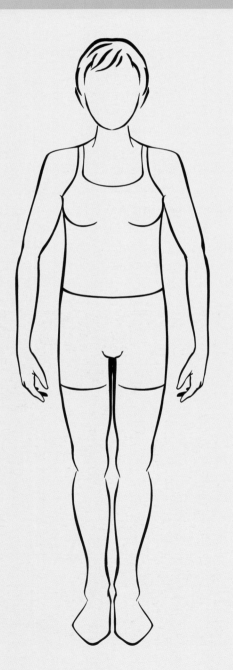

- Your body is hard and muscular.
- You have a straight up and down shape.
- Your overall frame is somewhat short and chunky.
- You are able to eat lots, yet your body weight does not fluctuate much.
- Your joints are strong.
- You have excellent circulation.
- You have a low heart rate.
- Your strength is excellent.
- You have poor flexibility.
- You are very athletic.

However, your body frame can be somewhat chunky and masculine and also inflexible. Our overall goal will be to make you more supple and less bulky.

The Pencil Shape

The perfect supermodel shape? Your frame is ideally suited to the catwalk, but often your posture is not good and your muscle tone is poor. You find it very hard to build muscle no matter how much strength work you do, yet you are very good at sports that require stamina, running the marathon for example.

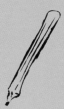

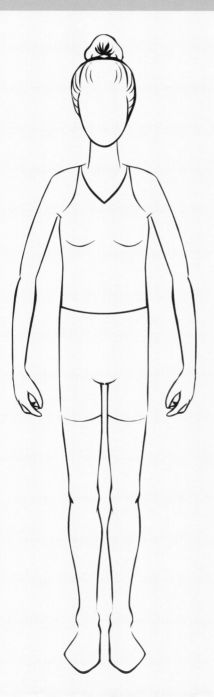

- You are usually tall and thin.
- You have a fragile frame.
- Your high metabolic rate means you can eat lots without gaining weight.
- Your limbs are slender.
- You have narrow shoulders and hips.
- You are small-boned.
- You are very lightly muscled.
- Your cardiovascular system is poor.
- You have a high heart rate.
- You have floppy, often unstable joints.
- You have poor muscle endurance.
- Your strength is poor.

However, just to confuse you, there is every chance you are a mixture of different body shapes, so don't worry if it's too difficult to pinpoint your exact shape. Decide instead which area of your body you need to work on. The exercises have been grouped by the body area they affect most, so you can design your own workouts regardless of body shape.

The more you learn about your body the better equipped you will be to design your fitness routine. When you have determined your body shape and read through the recommendations below, work out your Body Mass Index (BMI) (page 23) before you start the programme and check it again at the end of four weeks; it will help indicate how you are progressing.

The Pear-Shaped Programme

Your priorities are to lose fat and build more muscle,
to improve your BMI and tone your problem areas.

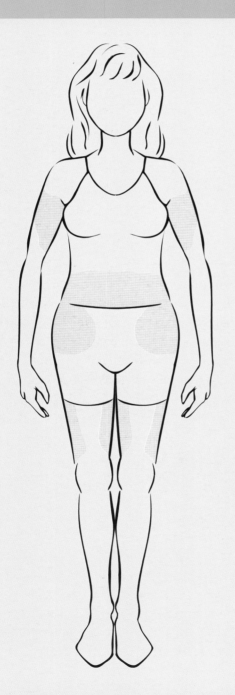

Your problem aras are:

abdominals
upper arms
inner thighs
outer thighs
hips
buttocks

Strength training is very important for you, and fortunately there are many different ways you can build muscle. One option is to do exercises which use hand and leg weights, such as the Axe (page 116), which help sculpt your upper arms, and Boxes Abduction and Circles Adduction (pages 86–8), which help trim your outer and inner thighs. When you first attempt these exercises always start with the lightest weights recommended, but once you've mastered the technique progress to using heavier weights. Alternatively, you can include exercises in your workout which use your body's weight against gravity to increase muscle tone such as One-Arm Push Ups (page 118), abdominal exercises such as Curl Ups with Frog's Legs (page 95), New Cancan (page 98) and Spine Curls with Arm Circles (page 80).

To trim your hips and buttocks we have given you some amazing exercises such as Oyster 1 and 2 (page 84), Star Test (page 83) and Star Variation (page 108). You will find the Bottom Worker (page 82) very hard to do, so we have left it until the last two weeks of the programme. Omit it if you find it too difficult.

To shape your legs try the Leg Shaper (page 76).

Because you are bottom heavy, in addition to slimming down the hips it is worth developing the upper body to get a more even balance from top to bottom, which will help you achieve a more hourglass figure. Exercises such as Side Twist (page 114) and Boxing (page 117) will all help.

If you are going to lose fat you will need to do some aerobic exercise in addition to Pilates. Cardiovascular activity strengthens the heart and lungs and enhances your body's ability to transport oxygen, which is needed by the body to burn calories and fat. Brisk walking, cycling or swimming are all good forms of aerobic exercise (see page 24 for General Guidelines on Aerobic Exercise). Choose something you enjoy and which fits in easily with your schedule.

Exercises for pear shapes are indicated by
Please remember that although you need to focus in particular on these areas:

- strengthening abdominals
- sculpting upper arms
- toning inner/outer thighs
- streamlining hips
- firming buttocks
- improving posture

you also need to add other exercises to the programme for balance. We have done this for you in the workouts given on pages 124–6.

The Apple-Shaped Programme

Your priorities are to lose fat and build more muscle, to improve your BMI and tone your problem areas – in particular, the waist.

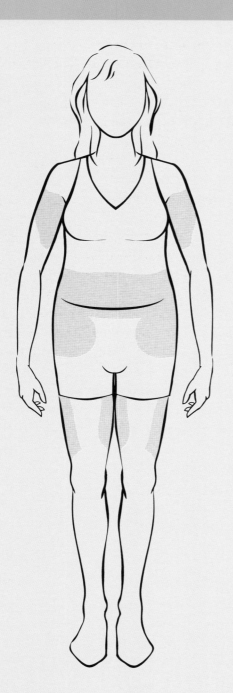

Your problem areas are:

abdominals
waist
upper arms
hips
buttocks
inner thighs
outer thighs

For the reasons already explained you are more prone to heart conditions so it is vital you include some extra cardiovascular work in your programme. Choose something you enjoy and which fits in easily with your schedule. (See the list of aerobic activities on page 24.)

To help change your apple shape we need to include plenty of abdominal and waist exercises: Oblique Roll Ups (page 97), Hip Rolls Variation (page 96) and Side Twist (page 114) are all good for you.

Another problem area can be the upper arms, so any exercises which require you to use your upper body are great: One-Arm Push Ups (page 118) will work your arms and your pectoral muscles, Stretching Mermaid (page 119) will do the same, while Axe (page 116) and Boxing (page 117) will help sculpt the arms.

You will be amazed at how exercises like Boxes Abduction (page 86) and Circles Adduction (page 88) work both your outer and inner thigh muscles, your buttocks and your waist muscles (just place your hand on your waist and feel the muscles working to keep your trunk still while the legs move). The Leg Shaper (page 76) will also help shape your legs.

To tone your buttocks try Spine Curls with Arm Circles (page 80), Bottom Worker (page 82), Oyster 1 and 2 (page 84) and Star Variation (page 108).

Exercises for apple shapes are indicated by 🍎
Please remember that although you need to focus particularly on these areas:
• strengthening abdominals
• streamlining the waist
• sculpting upper arms
• trimming hips
• firming buttocks
• toning inner/outer thighs
• improving posture

you should also add other exercises to the programme for balance. The exercises for your particular problem areas are identical to those in the Pear-Shaped Programme. However, the actual workouts (pages 127–9) we have created for you have many more abdominal and waist exercises than the programme for pear shapes.

Body Shapes

17

The Rectangular-Shaped Programme

You have the ideal athletic frame but, although sport and fitness comes easily to you, there are still areas for improvement. You are naturally muscular, but you need to balance this with flexibility training.

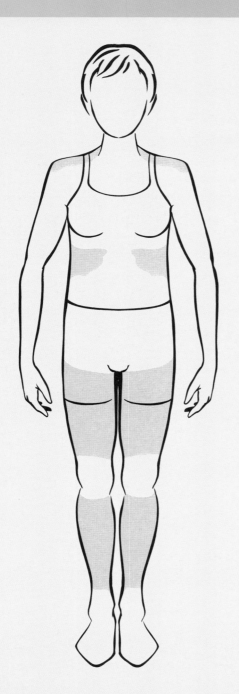

Your problem areas are:

tight upper shoulders
tight upper abdominals
tight front/back/inner thighs and calves

We will be aiming to give you a good workout yet at the same time ensure you do not over-train. Make sure you always include stretches in your workout – yes, even those stretches you don't like!

Pilates stretches are often part of a movement such as those in Leg Sweeps (page 78). This is a dynamic or moving stretch, where one muscle stretches its opposing muscle during the movement. In this case the hip flexors and the quadriceps at the front of the thigh dynamically stretch the hamstrings at the back of the thigh as the leg is extended. These types of stretches are ideal for rectangular-shaped people and you will enjoy them more than static stretching where no movement is involved.

Other wonderful stretches for you include Side Twist (page 114), Threading a Needle with Arm Openings (page 115), Stretching Mermaid (page 119) and Upright Chair Stretch (page 92). You may not find these stretches easy at first, but your body will gradually become more supple as you practise Pilates regularly.

Try to avoid overtraining, especially weight training, because this will bulk up your muscles, shortening rather than lengthening them. This does not mean you should not use weights, but you should be careful not to overuse them. Pilates is perfect for you because you will develop long, strong muscles rather than short, strong muscles. Take your time and work slowly, with control, to ensure good technique.

Exercises which work the whole body are the best way forward because they maintain the balance of the body and avoid one area becoming overdeveloped.

If you have built up your muscles at the gym, remember that your superficial muscles, the ones you can see, need to be supported by deep postural muscles to ensure good movement patterns and to avoid joint problems. This is why we have prescribed lots of stability exercises such as Knee Folds (page 48), Oyster 1 and 2 (page 84), Leg Sweeps (page 78) and Star Variation (page 108). You must do these exercises slowly and precisely. You may feel they are too easy for you but it is essential you do the basic stability work on pages 40–64. Having worked over the years with many top athletes, we have discovered they think they can do these exercises well, but in fact they are usually cheating! So slow down and focus.

Include any aerobic activity that you enjoy in your weekly regime, but do not overdo it.

Allow time for relaxation. Massage is great for everyone, but especially good for you. That's official!

Exercises for rectangular shapes are indicated by ☐

Please remember that although you need to focus particularly on these areas:
- improving flexibility with lots of stretches
- building core stability to support your superficial muscles
- 'total body' exercises to restore the balance of your body
- improving the mobility of the spine
- relaxation
- improving posture

you should also add other exercises to the programme for balance, and on pages 130–2 we have compiled some balanced workouts for you.

The Pencil-Shaped Programme

The elegant, graceful figure of the pencil-shaped woman is the envy of most of us. However, many very slim people have very poor muscle tone, very floppy joints and poor posture.

Your problem areas are:

rounded shoulders
tense neck
buttocks
thighs
upper arms
abdominals
calves

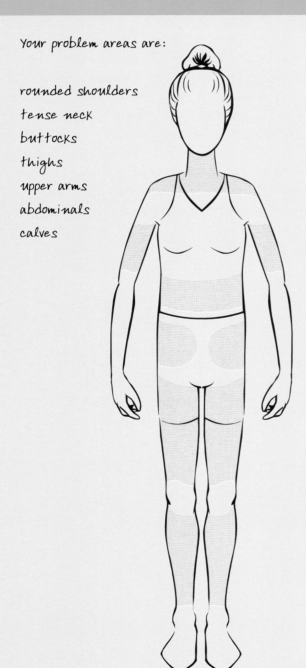

To improve your posture you need to do plenty of body-awareness exercises such as Starfish (pages 62 and 63), the standing exercises (pages 67–9) and Cleopatra (page 72). To prevent round shoulders the Diamond Press Salute (page 107) and the Dart (page 56) are great for you.

You should concentrate on gaining weight in the form of lean muscle tissue, but you need to be careful not to do too much too quickly; build muscle slowly. Because your frame is so slight, bulky muscle would look very unflattering. Little and often is the best way forward. Using the body's own weight against gravity with exercises such as One-Arm Push Ups (page 118) is useful but, because you are light, these sort of exercises need to be supplemented with extra strength training using weights. You should use light to medium weights with exercises such as Boxing (page 117) and the Axe (page 116).

As you can suffer from unstable joints, you must also include plenty of stability work. This is why we have added the Pelvic Stability Exercises (pages 45–52) from the Basics of Body Control Pilates chapter to your programme.

You can try to add curves to your straight up and down shape by choosing exercises that sculpt the buttocks, legs, shoulders and arms. Good exercises for your buttocks include Spine Curls (page 80), Bottom Worker (page 82), Oyster 1 and 2 (page 84), Boxes Abduction (page 86) and Circles Adduction (page 88).

Pencil-shaped people often have poorly aligned and weak legs and the Leg Shaper (page 76) is a good exercise to help correct this.

Exercises that work your abdominals and define your waist will also give you a more hourglass curvy shape if that's what you wish for. Curl Ups with Frog's Legs (page 95) and New Cancan (page 98) are all good for this. Hip Rolls Variation (page 96) is great for trimming the waist, as is Oblique Roll Ups (page 97). Stretching Mermaid (page 119) is also good for both stretching and working the waist.

You must include some cardiovascular activities to keep your heart healthy. Avoid heavy training sessions as they may be counter-productive, putting stress and strain on your joints. Choose activities you enjoy. Your body type makes you naturally good at distance running or walking, less good at ball sports or any activity that requires bursts of speed or strength.

Pencil-shaped people can be prone to a rather nervous disposition, so be sure to include some relaxation time in your week. Pilates breathing can help you unwind. By using the breath to control your movements, you can learn to release tension and de-stress.

Exercises for pencil shapes are indicated by
Please remember that although you need to focus particularly on these areas:
- improving all-over muscle tone
- improving joint stability
- improving posture
- gentle weight work
- sculpting buttocks, arms and shoulders
- defining waistline
- shaping legs
- releasing tension with breath control

you should also add other exercises to the programme for balance, and on pages 133–5 we have compiled some balanced workouts for you.

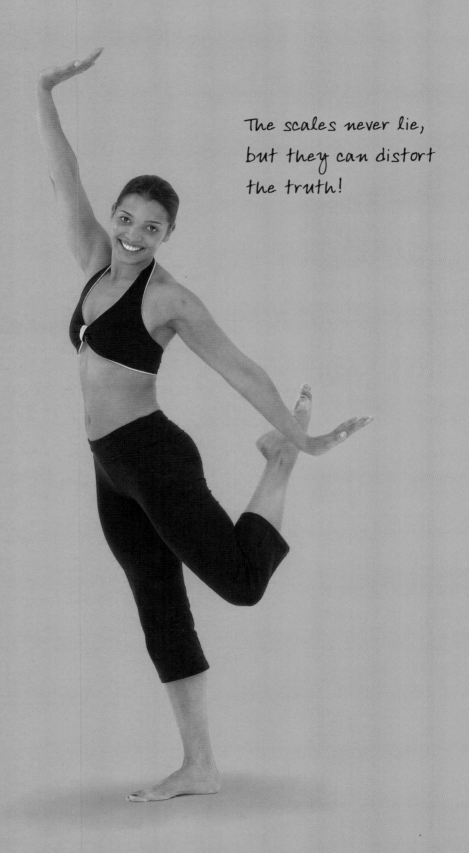

The Complete Picture

The scales never lie,
but they can distort
the truth!

Body Mass Index (BMI)

Whatever shape you are, you should take a few moments to work out your BMI.

It is quite possible for someone to be within the ideal weight range, as determined by a weight for height chart, yet still be carrying too much fat, as is sometimes the case for pencil shapes. Equally, because muscle is heavier than fat, a very muscular person, a rectangular shape, may appear overweight as judged by the same charts.

BMI is a more accurate predictor of the health risks associated with being over- or underweight than weight alone. There is a wealth of scientific evidence that suggests a BMI between 18.5 and 25 is associated with the lowest health risks. But the risks increase slightly below 18.5, increase significantly above 25 and increase dramatically with a BMI over 30. Although BMI alone does not give you information about body fat, using it in conjunction with waist circumference will give you a better idea. If your BMI is above 25 and your waist circumference is above 89 cm for women and 102 cm for men, it suggests that the excess weight you are carrying is fat and not muscle.

How You Shape Up

You can work out your BMI using this simple equation:

$$BMI = \frac{\text{your weight (in kilos)}}{\text{your height (in metres squared)}}$$

For example $\dfrac{60 \text{ kg}}{(1.65 \text{ m} \times 1.65 \text{ m})} = 22$

(1 kg = 2.2 lb: 1 m = 39.37 in)

18.5–25 is acceptable
25–30 is overweight
30–40 is obese
over 40 is severely obese

Waist Circumference

You need to lose weight if your waist circumference measures:

over 102 cm for men
over 89 cm for women

General Guidelines for Aerobic Exercise

- Have a check-up with a doctor before embarking on any cardiovascular exercise programme.

- If the situation permits, use a heart-rate monitor where possible (they are very easy to use). Exercising at the correct intensity is essential to ensure safe and effective training. The American College of Sports Medicine recommends an exercise intensity of between 60 to 90 per cent of maximum predicted heart rate (220 minus your age), based on healthy individuals. This is quite complex, and a much simpler way to judge if you have the right intensity is the talk test. In a nutshell, if you cannot hold a light conversation while you are exercising because you are breathless, then you are working too hard.

- Do not go too fast too soon. Build your fitness steadily and progressively. Work at your own level. If you have a low level of aerobic fitness, start with moderate exercise such as walking, stationary cycling or swimming.

- As your aerobic fitness improves, increase the duration and intensity of your training while still monitoring your heart rate.

- Avoid carrying unnecessary tension especially in your shoulders; relax and monitor your breathing.

- Avoid overtraining one area of the body by varying your activities.

- Government guidelines recommend 5 x 30 minutes of aerobic activity a week for a healthy heart. This does not have to be done all at once, it can be accumulative, that is, you can do 3 x 10 minute sessions a day. This is not as hard as it sounds, for example, a brisk walk to the station in the mornings, another brisk walk at lunchtime and then a brisk walk home back from the station all adds up. This is the bare minimum you need to do to keep your heart healthy. However, to build your overall fitness level and to help you tone up, you should consider adding to this other cardiovascular activities (see recommended list and guidelines below).

- Longer continuous cardiovascular sessions. Because we are going for a complete change of shape within four weeks, pear and apple shapes, who need to burn more fat, will have to increase the amount of aerobic work to burn more calories. In addition to the 3 x 10 minutes a day, you must also do a minimum of two sessions of 30 consecutive minutes of aerobic activity a week. Choose an activity or class to suit your body type, level of fitness, physical limitations and needs. Good choices are:

    - jogging (treadmill or outdoors)
    - swimming
    - cycling (stationary or outdoors)
    - rollerblading
    - spinning (instructor-led class)
    - kick boxing
    - aerobics class
    - cross trainer (machine)
    - rowing (indoors or outdoors)
    - dancing

- Ensure you are using the correct footwear for your chosen activity. Incorrect footwear can lead to conditions such as shin splints and ankle injuries.

- Consider purchasing a pedometer, which measures the number of steps you take in a day. You should aim to do 10,000 steps a day to stay fit, healthy and to manage your weight.

Weight Management

It would be remiss of us not to mention diet in a book that promises a new body. Good nutrition is an essential part of achieving a healthy fit body.

Pilates is not a weight-loss programme; however, as you build more muscle into your body you improve your BMI and are better able to control your weight. Please remember that we are all individual and have different needs. Pear and apple shapes will have to manage their weight in a different way to pencil shapes (where being underweight is often an issue). This is why we prefer the term weight management to weight loss.

There is no mystery as to why we gain weight; it's a simple equation. We gain weight when the energy (calories) we consume exceeds the energy we use. In this situation, excess energy is stored in the body as fat. Eating a small amount in excess of your needs will result in a slow but steady weight gain. Eating just 100 calories a day more than you need, the equivalent of one and a half digestive biscuits, will result in weight gain of 4.7 kg (10 lb) in a year.

There are many fad diets around at the moment, some, such as the Atkins Diet, have unleashed a great deal of controversy. Because of such controversy, we recommend you eat a sensible, balanced, low-fat, calorie-restricted diet. To lose weight you simply need to tip the balance so you use more calories than you consume. You can do this either by restricting the number of calories you eat or by increasing the amount of calories you use, but without doubt the best way is a combination of diet and exercise.

For more information on a healthy balanced diet please consult two of our earlier books *Pilates Plus Diet* (Pan) or *The Perfect Body the Pilates Way* (Pan).

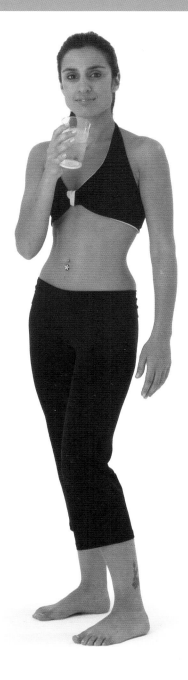

The Complete Picture

25

Devising Your Own Workouts

If you feel confident, in addition to the workouts we have designed for you, you can of course create your own sessions. You may have learnt other Pilates exercises elsewhere and these can be included. Vary your workouts, not forgetting to include those exercises recommended for your body type. In fact, most Pilates exercises work the entire body simultaneously – that's one of our secrets. However, if you are worried about a particular area you can include more repetitions of an exercise if you wish, but take care not to unbalance your body.

When you are devising your own workouts, try to maintain the balance by including the following spinal movements:

flexion (bending forward)

– for example, Curl Ups with Frog's Legs (page 95)

rotation (twisting)

– for example, Hip Rolls Variation, Threading a Needle (pages 96, 115)

extension (bending backward)

– for example, Diamond Press Salute (page 107)

lateral flexion (bending sideways)

– for example, Side Twist, Stretching Mermaid (pages 114, 119)

Then add a balance of upper-and-lower body work, stretching and weight work.

The Eight Principles of Body Control Pilates

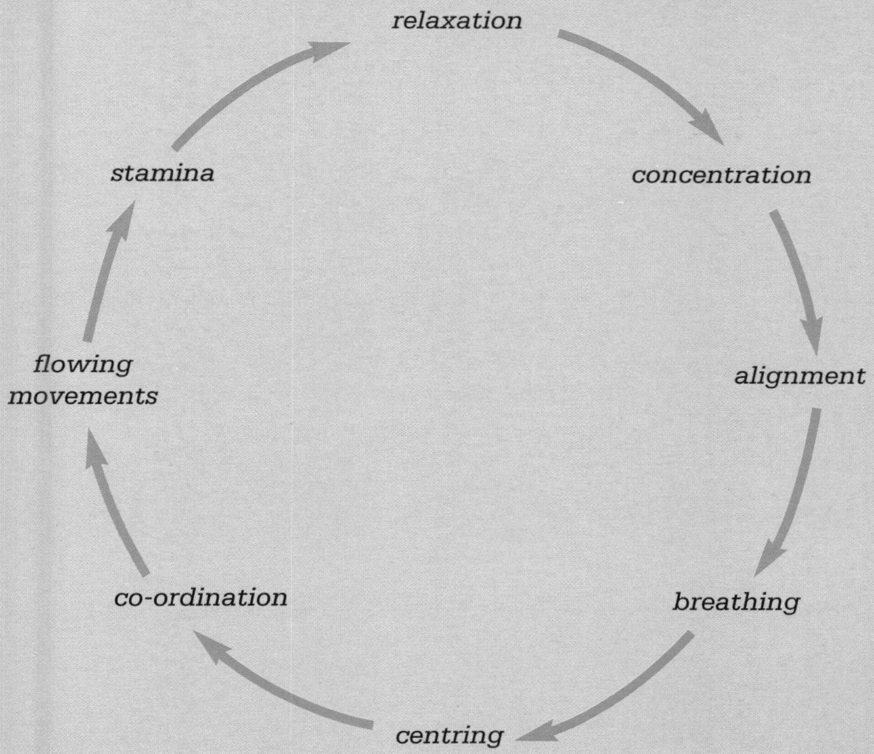
relaxation
concentration
alignment
breathing
centring
co-ordination
flowing movements
stamina

Relaxation

The recognition and release of unwanted tension in the body is the starting point for our teaching.

Concentration

Hand in hand with relaxation goes concentration.

Next time you feel yourself under pressure, stop and take note of which parts of your body are tense – your jaw, neck, shoulders, back? It is often very hard for these muscles to release, so they stay continually switched on.

One of our first priorities is, therefore, to help you learn how to switch them off, otherwise they can remain dominant and prevent natural movement. But by relaxed we do not mean collapsed; we need you ready to exercise, to move freely using the right muscles to make the movements.

The Relaxation Position on page 34 is a good way to start a session and you will also notice that we use it as the starting and finishing position for many of the exercises.

Pilates is a mental and physical conditioning programme that should help train both your mind and your body. Because it requires you to focus on each movement made, it develops your body's sensory feedback, or proprioception, so you know where you are in space and what you are doing with every part of your body for every second you are moving. Although the movements themselves may become automatic with time, you still have to concentrate because there is always a further level of awareness to reach.

Use the exercises in this book to improve your mind/body connection and you will find that you are far more body aware, not just when you exercise but also in your daily activities. You will be able to concentrate better and will be far more co-ordinated in your movements. Learn to listen to the natural intelligence of your body – it really does talk to you!

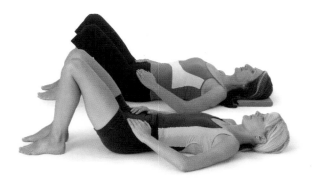

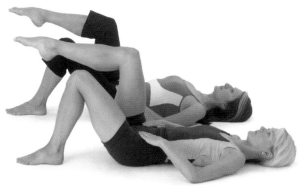

Alignment

Good postural alignment is at the centre of our technique.

Alignment is essential not only for restoring muscle balance, good body mechanics and preventing aches and pains but also to help you look good. If you exercise without concern for the correct position of the bones and joints, you risk stressing them, which can lead to extra wear and tear.

Muscles have an optimal length at which they function best; if you have poor postural alignment this length may be held altered, and the muscles can end up too long or too short; either way their ability to do their job properly is affected and poor muscle recruitment is the result. By placing your bones in the right alignment before you start an exercise and being aware of where they are while you do the exercise, you stand a better chance of getting the right muscles working, resulting in good movement patterns, which means your workout is going to be really effective.

What we are aiming for is for you to be able to recognize and keep your joints in their 'neutral' positions, which is the ideal position for good muscle balance and healthy ligaments. Gradually your body will 'remember' the positions and you will find yourself sitting correctly and walking taller.

Many of our exercises require you to have your spine and pelvis in their natural neutral positions. For the spine, this means the position where it keeps its length and its natural S shape. This is the position where there is least stress on the facet joints, the ligaments and the discs and which allows the muscles to be at their optimal length and so function normally when we move. The Compass on page 35 is designed to help you find the correct natural neutral position of the pelvis and the spine.

Please remember that good alignment refers to the whole body. How you place your hands, feet, head, neck and shoulders while doing the exercises will all contribute to good posture. Pay close attention to the directions given in each exercise. A misplaced foot may prevent your pelvis from being in neutral; a tilted head can cause muscle tension.

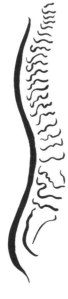

Neutral Spine

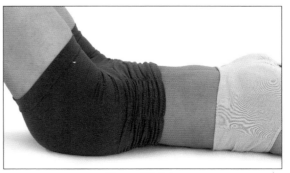

Neutral Pelvis

Breathing

Before any real benefit can be derived from physical exercises, one must first learn how to breathe properly. Our very life depends on it. – Joseph Pilates

Improving your breathing is probably the single most dramatic difference you can make to your overall health, but it is the one thing we all take for granted. Few of us breathe efficiently, and what a waste that is because we are missing out on all that wonderful oxygen which nourishes and replenishes every cell in the body and has an important role to play in burning calories and shedding fat.

The Pilates method teaches lateral thoracic breathing using the lower and the upper lobes of the lungs. You will learn how to use your breath to control your movements and release tension. By taking the time to learn Pilates breathing you can improve your overall well-being. What's more, once this breathing becomes automatic, once it becomes your natural unconscious way of breathing, you reap its benefits every second of the day and night.

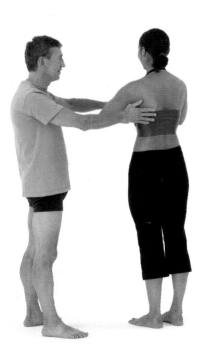

Centring: Creating a 'Girdle of Strength'

Joseph Pilates discovered that if he hollowed his navel back towards his spine, his low back felt protected and thus he introduced the direction 'navel to spine' for all his exercises. He called the area between the hips and the ribcage 'the powerhouse' and taught that all movements should originate from this strong centre, this natural 'girdle of strength'. In so doing he was using his deep postural muscles – transversus abdominis, the deepest of your abdominal muscles, and multifidus, a deep spinal muscle – to stabilize his spine, which modern physiotherapists now call core stability.

If you think of the vertebrae of your spine being like a pile of books stacked on top of each other, the role of transversus and multifidus is to prevent one of the books slipping out of place. In other words, they prevent one vertebra from slipping too far off its neighbour resulting in everything from facet-joint to disc problems. Unfortunately, poor posture often means that the deep stabilizing muscles are held lengthened and thus weakened.

The exercises on pages 41–4 will teach you how to locate and strengthen your deep stabilizing muscles with the 'zip up and hollow' action.

Once you have learned to create a strong centre, you can start to challenge that stability by moving your limbs and adding spinal movements such as rotation, flexion, lateral flexion and extension. A good workout should include all these movements.

What we are aiming for is free-flowing movements around a strong base. Bear in mind that all the joints in the body have stabilizing muscles whose role it is to fix and hold the bones in good alignment to allow the more superficial (mobilizing) muscles to execute the movements. When these deep stabilizing muscles are weak, perhaps as a result of poor posture, the balance of the muscles is upset and the more superficial mobilizing muscles have to take on the stabilizing role.

Co-ordination

So now you are relaxed, focused, aware, aligned, you are breathing efficiently (or learning to) and you have located and strengthened your deep core muscles.

For example, if your hamstrings are really tight despite a lot of stretching, it may be that they are shortened because they are having to stabilize the pelvis. This may be due to the fact that the muscles which should stabilize the pelvis – transversus abdominis and the deep gluteals (buttock muscles) – are weak. Similarly, if your low back feels tight, it may be that the erector spinae muscle group (primarily mobilizing muscles) are having to do the work that the deep stabilizing muscles (transversus and multifidus) are not doing properly.

If your stabilizing muscles are weak, your movement patterns will be upset and your joints placed under strain. This is why we aim to build strength from the inside out. First we must learn how to position the body correctly, then we need to strengthen the deep postural muscles. Once we have done this, we can learn good movement skills and then go on to strengthen the rest of the body.

Now you are ready to add movement. Step by step, the exercises teach you how to move well. It may seem strange to begin with, it will feel different (after all, you have probably been moving badly for many years), but the movements soon become automatic, ingrained or 'grooved' as they are locked into the body's memory. Meanwhile, the actual process of learning these new co-ordination skills is excellent mental and physical training, stimulating the two-way communication channel between mind and body.

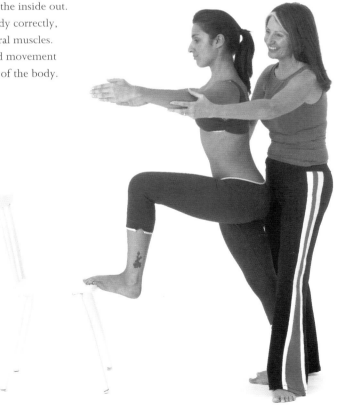

The Eight Principles of Body Control Pilates

Flowing Movements

Pilates is about natural movements performed smoothly, gracefully and with attention to detail.

Stamina

Stamina is going to be both a goal and an end result of your hard endeavours.

You will not be required to twist into awkward positions or to strain. We start with small movements and build up to more complicated combinations; the idea is to be constantly challenged. As beginners, you need to keep your limbs close to you, rather than risk losing your alignment and stability, but as you grow more confident and proficient you will take your joints through their full range of motion. Whatever exercise you perform, the movements must be precisely executed with control. The movements are generally slow, lengthening away from a strong centre, which gives you the opportunity to check your alignment and focus on using the right muscles. Slow doesn't mean easy though, in fact it is harder to do an exercise slowly than quickly, and it is also less easy to cheat!

Tiredness and lack of energy seem to be commonplace these days. Poor health can often be a cause, but it is worth remembering that poor posture and bad movement patterns may contribute to tiredness. Standing badly is tiring: the ribcage is compressed and, as a consequence, the lungs are constricted. As you learn to open and lengthen the body, your breathing becomes more efficient. All Pilates exercises are designed to encourage the respiratory, lymphatic and circulatory systems to function more effectively. As you become more proficient at the exercises and your muscles begin to strengthen and work correctly, you will discover that your overall stamina improves dramatically. You will no longer be wasting energy holding on to unnecessary tension or moving inefficiently, your body will move as nature intended.

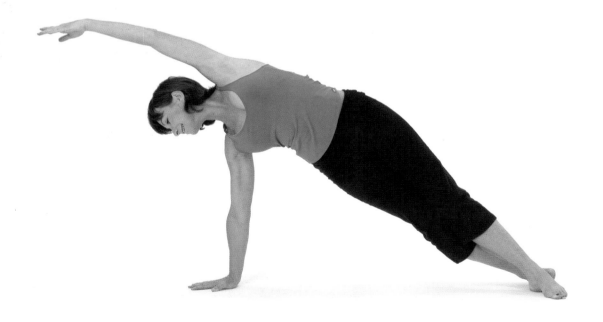

Step by step we are going to teach you the basic skills you need to perform the exercises well. Once you have mastered one skill you can move on to the next. You will find that learning one skill helps with learning the others. At first you will find keeping neutral, breathing wide, zipping up and hollowing difficult to do simultaneously, but it will all come together and then you can move on. The basic skills are good alignment, breathing and centring.

The Basics of Body Control Pilates

Alignment

Relaxation Position

One of the easiest ways to find good alignment is through an exercise we call the Relaxation Position. It is used as a starting and finishing position for many of our exercises.

1 Lie on your back with a folded towel or firm, flat pillow underneath your head if necessary, to allow the back of the neck to lengthen.
2 Have your knees bent and keep your feet firmly on the floor, parallel and hip-distance apart, that is, in a line with the centre of your buttocks.
3 Put your hands on your lower abdomen (you may need to put your hands by your sides if using the Relaxation Position as a starting position).

Run through a checklist. Ask yourself:
• Am I holding tension in my neck and shoulders? Allow your neck to soften and your shoulders to widen and melt into the mat.
• Does my low back feel tight? Check you have kept the natural curves of your spine, then allow the spine to lengthen.
• Is my pelvis level? Is my sacrum square on the mat? (See the Compass opposite.)
• Are my thighs tense? Adjust your feet. Bring them nearer to your bottom or take them further away.
• Have I got my knees in a line with my hips? Try lining them up with the middle of each buttock cheek.
• Can I feel the three points on the soles of my feet in contact with the floor: base of the big toes, base of the small toes, centre of the heels?

When you have completed your checklist, you can begin the exercise confident that your alignment is good and you have let go of any unnecessary tension. Remain vigilant while you perform the exercises or those overactive, dominant muscles will kick back in.

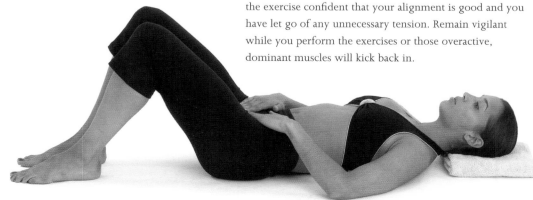

Compass – Finding Neutral

To achieve good body alignment you need to recognize when your pelvis and spine are in their natural neutral positions and you then need to develop the strength to maintain this. The angle of your pelvis affects the angle of your spine, so learning how to find your neutral pelvis is the first step towards finding your neutral spinal position.

1 Lie in the Relaxation Position (opposite).

2 Imagine you have a compass on your lower abdomen. The navel is north and the pubic bone south, with west and east on either side. Now try two incorrect positions in order to find the correct one.

3 Tilt your pelvis north. The pelvis will tuck under, the waist will flatten and the curve of the lower back is lost as your tailbone lifts off the mat. You will also grip your abdominals.

4 Next, carefully and gently move the pelvis in the other direction so that it tilts south; don't go too far, just a little way. (Avoid this bit if you have a back injury.) The low back will arch, the ribs will flare and the stomach sticks out. Come back to the Relaxation Position.

5 Aim for a neutral position between these two extremes. Go back to the image of the compass and think of the pointer as a spirit level. When you are in neutral, the pubic bone and pelvic bones will be level north, south, east and west. Your sacrum will rest squarely on the mat and you should feel as though the tailbone is lengthening away along the mat. Try also to keep both sides of the waist long and equal.

6 Now bring your awareness to your spine. Think of the 'S' shape of the spine. Think of lengthening through the spine while keeping those natural curves.

Once you are familiar with neutral in the Relaxation Position, you should practise finding it while standing, sitting and lying on your side so that it becomes normal. Please note that if the muscles around the pelvis are very out of balance, you may find neutral difficult to maintain. When this is the case, it is often necessary to work in what is the best neutral you can achieve or use support such as towels or flat pillows. Usually, after a few months, as the muscles begin to rebalance, neutral becomes more comfortable.

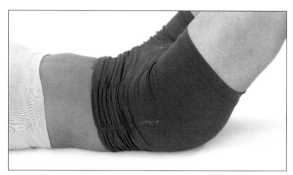

North

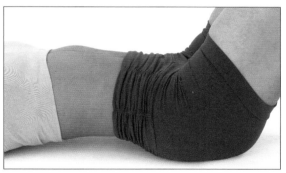

South

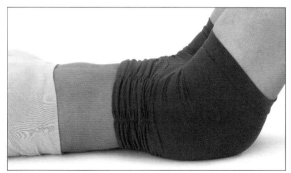

Neutral Pelvis

Standing Alignment

Knee–Foot Alignment

For good standing alignment, see the standing exercises on pages 67–9

The knees should be kept in a line with the second toe in all activities even when the leg is turned out from the hip. Whenever the knees are bent in a standing position, they should go directly over the second toes.

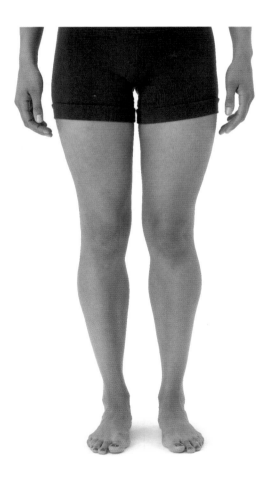

Side-Lying Alignment

Lie on your side in a straight line. It helps to use the edge of your mat as a guide. Have your underneath arm stretched out in a line with your body with a small flat pillow between your ear and arm so your neck keeps in line with your spine. Bend your knees, keeping your feet in line with your bottom. Line your joints up: ankle over ankle; knee over knee; shoulder over shoulder. Your hips are square, not tilted forwards or backwards. Your waistline is lifted off the floor.

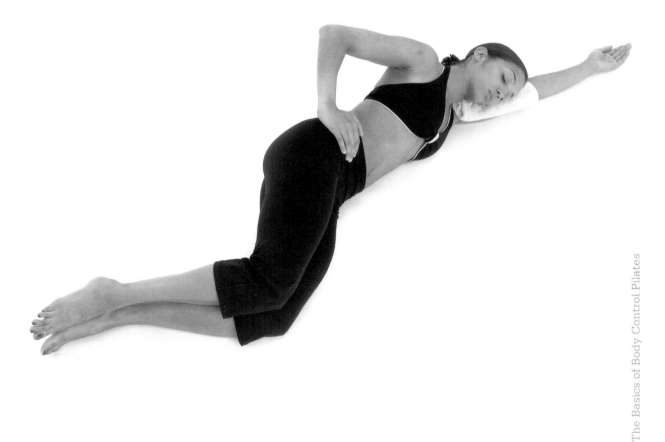

Prone Alignment

Four-Point Kneeling Alignment

Lie on your front in a straight line. You might be amazed how hard this is; most of us tend to lie at an angle. Have your feet hip-width apart and in parallel. Your pelvic bones and hip bones should rest evenly on the mat. If you are uncomfortable in this position, place a flat pillow or folded towel under your abdomen to support your lower back. Ultimately, you want to lie without this support. Depending on the exercise to be performed, you can either rest your head on your folded hands or have your arms down by your sides. If the latter, then place a folded towel or flat pillow under your forehead so your neck retains its natural curve and remains lengthened. The upper body should be open and a distance maintained between the ears and the shoulders.

For good four-point kneeling alignment, see page 42 Zipping on All Fours.

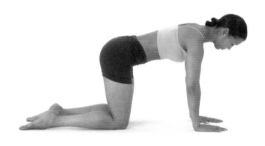

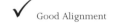
✓ Good Alignment

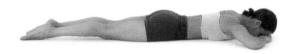

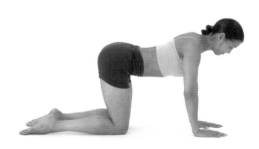
✗ Bad Alignment

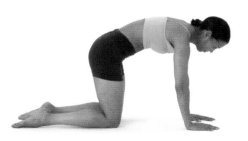
✗ Bad Alignment

Breathing

Stand in front of a mirror and watch as you take a deep breath.
Do your shoulders rise up around your ears or does your lower stomach
expand when you breathe in?

Most of us breathe inefficiently. Ideally, you should breathe wide and full into your back and sides. This makes sound sense because the lungs are situated in the ribcage and by expanding them, the volume of the cavity is increased and the capacity for oxygen intake is therefore increased as well. It also encourages maximum use of the lower part of the lungs.

This type of breathing – called thoracic or lateral breathing – makes the upper body more fluid and mobile. The lungs become like bellows, with the lower ribcage expanding wide as you breathe in and closing down as you breathe out. As you breathe in your diaphragm automatically descends, the aim is not to stop this but rather to focus on the movement to be widthways and into the back. The lungs are just like balloons and they need to expand in all directions as they fill with air. Unfortunately for most of us the balloons never get to be fully inflated! Learning how to breathe thoracically will change that.

Try this simple exercise:

1 Sit or stand tall (you will never be able to breathe well unless you lengthen up through the body – with bad posture your ribcage is compressed). Wrap a scarf or towel around your ribs, crossing it over at the front.

2 Holding the opposite ends of the scarf and pulling it tight gently, breathe in and allow your ribs to expand the towel (watch that you do not lift the breastbone too high). Think of the ribs opening like an umbrella.

3 As you breathe out, you may gently squeeze the towel to help fully empty your lungs and relax the ribcage, allowing the breastbone to soften. The umbrella closes.

Also important to Pilates is the timing of the breath. Most people find this timing difficult at first, especially if you are used to other fitness regimes, but once you have mastered it, it makes sense.

As a general rule:

• Breathe in to prepare for a movement.
• Breathe out, zip up and hollow (page 41), exhaling fully while you move.
• Breathe in, still zipped, to recover.
• Never hold your breath.

Moving on the exhalation will enable you to relax into the movement and prevent you from tensing. It also offers greater core stability at the hardest part of the exercise and safeguards against holding the breath, which can unduly stress the heart and lead to serious complications. Remember to focus on the out-breath completely - emptying the lungs. When you do this, the in-breath will naturally come flooding in.

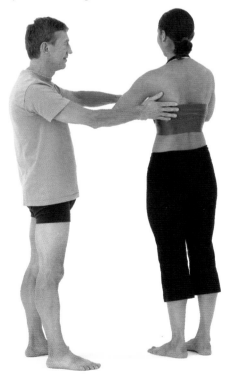

Centring: Core Strength

Now we need to locate and engage those all-important core stabilizing muscles: the pelvic floor, transversus abdominis and multifidus.

One of the most important aspects in all stability work is engaging the muscles at the right amount. Muscles can work from 0–100 per cent effort. Try standing up and tightening your buttocks as much as you can (100 per cent). Now try to release them about 50 per cent. Then let go half that again to 25 per cent – that's how much you should be working your deep muscles.

This is because these muscles have to work for you all day every day – if you work them harder they will fatigue when they need endurance. For basic stability work we want you to work the muscles gently at no more than 25 per cent. Of course when you are doing an advanced exercise such as Curled-Up Leg Beats on page 101, you will need to work harder to stay stable.

Joseph Pilates used the direction 'navel to spine' to create a strong centre. Modern research has shown that the best stability is to be had if you first engage the pelvic floor muscles then the lower abdominals (transversus abdominis). This makes sense. Think of your torso: it is like a cardboard box filled with bottles. If you wanted to carry that box safely would you support it only at the sides? You would hold it from underneath to give maximum stability. It's the same with the pelvic floor and transversus; it is better to use them in combination to ensure good stability. It is important to engage the pelvic floor muscles first, drawing them up inside until you feel the lower abdominals engage. This is the 'zip up and hollow'.

Let's just clarify where the pelvic floor muscles are. They run front to back underneath forming a hammock on which all your abdominal contents rest. For our exercises we need to isolate only parts of your pelvic floor and to do so in a particular way. Be warned, this isn't easy and requires a lot of patience, a lot of practice and a lot of concentration!

One way to help locate these muscles is to suck your thumb as you draw them up inside. It sounds crazy, but it is effective! You want to think about these muscles as if you are lifting up from behind (as if you are trying to prevent yourself from passing wind but without clenching the buttocks). The muscles lift from back to front and, as they lift up and forward, they also draw together side to side like a camera shutter closing!

Try this exercise for awareness of where you are working and how hard you should work:

Zip Up and Hollow

This exercise was created to isolate and engage the deep stabilizing muscles of the pelvis, pelvic floor and spine.

Once you have learnt to zip up and hollow you need to learn how to zip up in different positions.

Starting Position

Sit tall on an upright chair making sure you are sitting square, with the weight even on both buttocks.

Action

1 Breathe in wide and full into your back and sides, then lengthen up through the spine.

2 As you breathe out, draw up the muscles of your pelvic floor from back to front, as if preventing wind, lifting up through the vagina (ladies only) and then imagining you are slowing down the flow of water. Gentlemen, you may imagine that you are lifting your family jewels (privates!). Draw these muscles up inside as if you are doing up an internal zip. Only zip up halfway to your navel. You do not need to reach as high as the navel itself; the action is low and gentle. You should be able to feel your lower abdominals hollow and scoop. This is as far as you need to engage the muscles, for zip up and hollow.

3 Breathe in and hold the zip up and hollow.

4 Breathe out and release.

5 Repeat 6 times, working up to holding the zip for several breaths.

watchpoints

- Always engage from the pelvic floor upwards, never the other way round.
- Always zip up before you move, not after.
- Keep the action gentle; remember 25 per cent!
- Do not allow the buttock muscles to join in.
- Keep your jaw relaxed.
- Don't tense your shoulders.
- Try not to grip around your hips.
- Keep the pelvis and spine quite still.

If you find that you are having trouble breathing laterally while zipped, you may have zipped up too high.

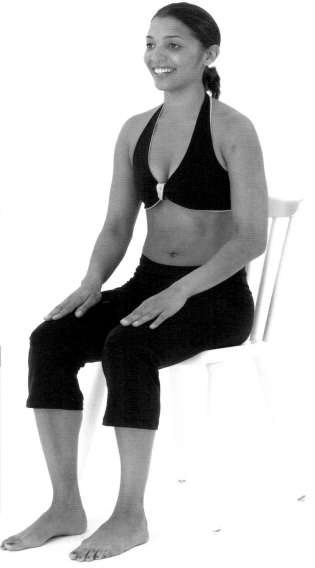

The Strong Zip

Zipping on All Fours

Try this wearing underwear, with a mirror underneath you. Check to see if your 'six-pack' (rectus abdominis) remains quiet! This is important, as it is a very dominant muscle.

For some of the more challenging exercises, such as Curled-Up Leg Beats on page 101 or New Cancan on page 98 you will need to zip up strongly. What do we mean by this? You can switch your zipping muscles on and off just like you turn on the volume on your stereo. It is very important that you always turn them on, that is engage them, gently to begin with or you risk the wrong muscles firing up. However, once they are 'switched on' it may be necessary to engage them more strongly like turning the volume up! This is fine. The secret is to engage slowly and gently to begin with and then to increase your zip only as much as you need to, no more.

watchpoints

- Check constantly that you are still breathing and that your ribcage is moving!
- Do not allow the pelvis to tuck under – stay neutral with your pelvis level.
- Do not push into the spine. Keep your tailbone lengthening away.

Starting Position

Kneel on all fours with your hands beneath your shoulders and your knees beneath your hips. Keep your elbows soft and directed backwards (this helps keep your shoulder blades down). Your spine should retain its natural curves. Have the top of your head lengthening away from your tailbone and your pelvis in neutral. Imagine a small pool of water resting at the base of your spine (it will help you to find neutral).

Action

1 Breathe in wide to prepare.
2 Breathe out, zip up from the pelvic floor and hollow the lower abdominals up and back towards the spine. Your back should not move. The pool of water stays put.
3 Breathe in and hold.
4 Breathe out and release.
5 Now try again, only this time add your lateral thoracic breathing and stay zipped while breathing in and out.
6 Repeat 6 times.

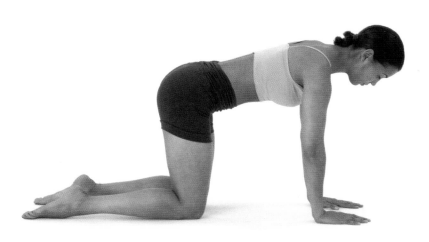

Zipping in Prone Lying

Starting Position

Lie face down, resting your head on your folded hands. Open the shoulders out and relax the upper back. Use a small, flat cushion under your abdomen if your low back is uncomfortable. Your legs are hip- or shoulder-distance apart and relaxed.

Action

1 Breathe in wide to prepare.
2 Breathe out, zip up from the pelvic floor and draw the lower abdominals back to your spine away from the floor.
3 Imagine there is a precious egg just above the pubic bone that must not be crushed. Do not tighten the buttocks – there should be no movement in the pelvis or the spine.
4 Breathe in and hold the zip.
5 Once again, try to stay zipped as you breathe in and out laterally.

Zipping in the Relaxation Position

Starting Position

Lie in the Relaxation Position (page 34). Find your hip bones (they are where your hipster jeans would sit). Place your fingers just inside these bones and feel that the lower abdominals are relaxed.

Action

1 Breathe in wide to prepare and lengthen through the spine.
2 Breathe out and zip up and hollow – your fingers should feel your abdominals engage. Breathe normally now as you keep these muscles working and try to think of them sinking back towards the spine. If they bulk up or go very tight you are working too hard.
3 Work up to keeping zipped for 5 breaths. Do not hold your breath.

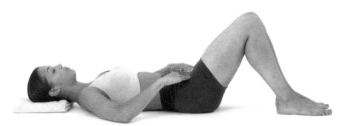

Zipping in Side-Lying

A useful preparation for all side-lying exercises.

Equipment

Two small pillows.

Starting Position

Lie on your side in a straight line. It helps to use the edge of your mat as a guide. Have your underneath arm stretched out in a line with your body with a small flat pillow between your ear and arm so your neck keeps in line with your spine. Bend your knees, keeping your feet in line with your bottom. Line your joints up: ankle over ankle; knee over knee; shoulder over shoulder. You can put a pillow between your knees to help keep the pelvis in a good position. Your hips are square, not tilted forwards or backwards. Your waistline is lifted off the floor.

Action

1 Breathe in wide and full and lengthen through the body.
2 Breathe out and gently zip up and hollow.
3 Stay zipped as you breathe normally for about 5 breaths. Do not allow your waist to sink into the floor. Keep lengthening through the body.

This, then, is your strong centre. For most of the exercises, you will be asked to zip up and hollow, drawing the lower abdominals back to the spine before and during your movements, lengthening away from a strong centre.

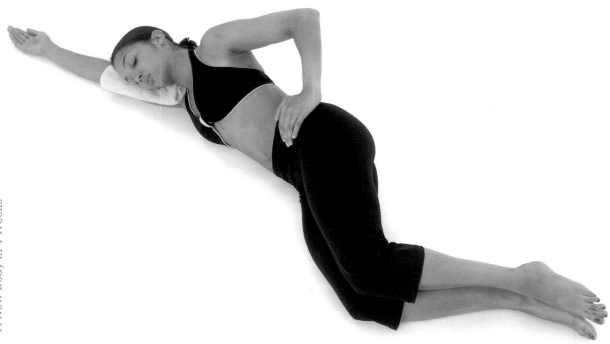

Having mastered breathing, correct alignment and the creation of a strong centre (zipping), you now need to learn how to add co-ordinated movements while keeping your core stability. It is not easy to begin with, but it soon becomes automatic. Meanwhile, the process of learning this co-ordination is fabulous mental and physical training as it stimulates that two-way communication between the brain and the muscles.

Start with small movements, then build up to more complicated combinations. Four movements to practise follow, all of them requiring you to keep the pelvis completely still. It might be useful to imagine that you have a set of car headlamps on your pelvis, shining at the ceiling. The beam should be fixed, not mimicking searchlights! You can vary which exercises you practise each session but the starting position is the same for all of them.

Remember: it is essential to zip up and hollow before you move.

Pelvic Stability Exercises

Leg Slides

Starting Position

Adopt the Relaxation Position (page 34). Check that your pelvis is in neutral, tailbone down and lengthening away, then place your hands on your hip bones to check for unwanted movement.

Action

1 Breathe in wide and full to prepare.
2 Breathe out, gently zip up and hollow, then slide one leg away along the floor in line with your hips. Keep the lower abdominals engaged and the pelvis still, stable and in neutral.
3 Breathe into your lower ribcage while you return the leg to the bent position, trying to keep the stomach hollow. If you cannot yet breathe in and maintain a strong centre, take an extra breath and return the leg on the out-breath.
4 Repeat 5 times with each leg.

watchpoints

- Remember that you are trying to avoid even the slightest movement of the pelvis. It helps to think of the waist being long and even on both sides as you make the movement.
- Try to keep your neck and jaw released throughout.
- Stay zipped and hollowed throughout.

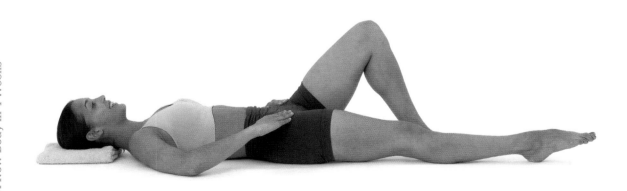

Knee Drops

Starting Position

As for Leg Slides.

Action

1 Breathe in wide and full to prepare.
2 Breathe out, gently zip up and hollow and allow one knee to open slowly to the side. Go only as far as the pelvis can stay still. It will want to roll side to side – don't let it.
3 Breathe in, staying zipped and hollowed as the knee returns to centre.
4   Repeat 5 times with each leg.

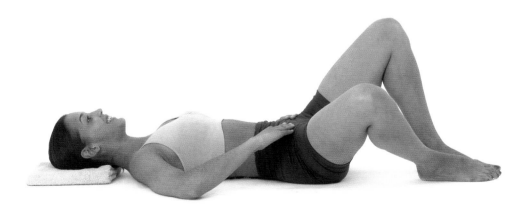

Knee Folds

This is a basic preparation for many Pilates abdominal exercises. With this movement it is particularly useful to feel that the muscles stay 'scooped' and do not bulge while you fold the knee in. Feel the muscles engage very gently as you zip up and hollow.

Starting Position

As for Leg Slides (page 46).

Action

1 Breathe in wide and full to prepare.
2 Breathe out, gently zip up and hollow, then fold one knee up. Think of the thighbone dropping down into the hip and anchoring there.
3 Do not lose your neutral pelvis – the tailbone stays down – and do not rely on the other leg to stabilize you. Imagine your foot is on a cream doughnut and you don't want to press down on it.
4 Breathe in and hold.
5 Breathe out, staying zipped and hollowed as you return the foot slowly to the floor.
6 Repeat 5 times with each leg.

As for Leg Slides (page 46).

watchpoints

- Remember that you are trying to avoid even the slightest movement of the pelvis. It helps to think of the waist being long and even on both sides as you make the movement.
- Try to keep your neck and jaw released throughout.
- Stay zipped and hollowed throughout.

If you find this very difficult you can bring your feet closer to you.

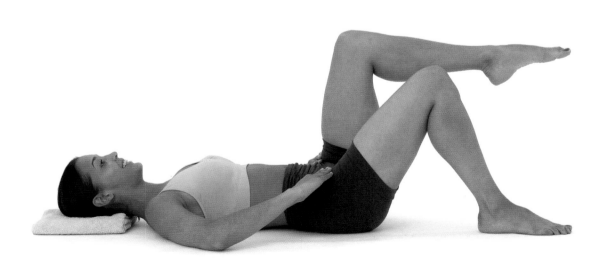

Knee Folds with Openings

Starting Position

As for Leg Slides (page 46).

Action

1 Breathe in wide and full to prepare.
2 Breathe out, gently zip up and hollow, and fold one knee up. Think of the thighbone dropping down into the hip and anchoring there. The shin of the folded leg should be parallel to the floor. Do not lose your neutral pelvis – the tailbone stays down – and do not rely on the other leg to stabilize you. Imagine your foot is on a cream doughnut and you don't want to press down on it.
3 Breathe in and hold.
4 Breathe out, still zipped and hollowed and take the whole leg out to the side to about 45 degrees (or as far as you can without losing neutral). The shin stays parallel to the floor.
5 Breathe in and bring the leg back to hip line.
6 Breathe out and slowly return the foot to the floor.
7 Repeat 5 times with each leg.

watchpoints

- Do not twist or tilt the pelvis as the leg moves to the side.
- Do not drop the foot.
- This is not a turn-out action (page 50).
- Do not hold your breath; use the breathing to help the movement.

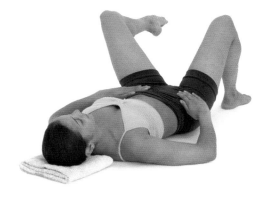

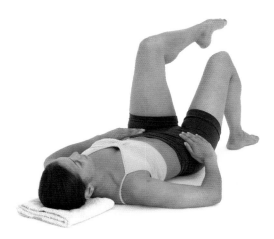

The Basics of Body Control Pilates

49

Turning Out the Leg

This next movement involves turning the leg out from the hip and is a preparation for exercises such as Pilates Stance (page 68) where the legs are held in a turned-out position. It works the deep gluteal muscles, especially gluteus medius, which is one of the main stabilizing muscles of the pelvis.

Starting Position

As for Leg Slides (page 46).

Action

1 Breathe in wide and full to prepare.
2 Breathe out, gently zip up and hollow, then fold the left knee up. Think of the thighbone dropping down into the hip and anchoring there.
3 Breathe in then out and, keeping zipped and hollowed, turn the left leg out from the hip bringing the left foot to touch the right knee if possible. Keep the knee in a line with the hip.
4 Do not allow the pelvis to tilt or twist or turn, keep it central and stable. (Headlamps glued to the ceiling!)
5 Breathe in, as you reverse the movement to return the foot to the floor.
6 Repeat 5 times on each side.

Please take advice if you suffer from sciatica.

watchpoints

- Remember that you are trying to avoid even the slightest movement of the pelvis. It helps to think of the waist being long and even on both sides as you make the movement.
- Try to keep your neck and jaw released throughout.
- Stay zipped and hollowed throughout.

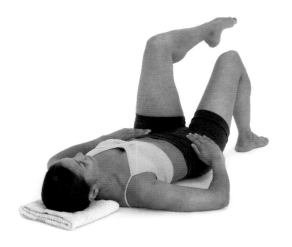
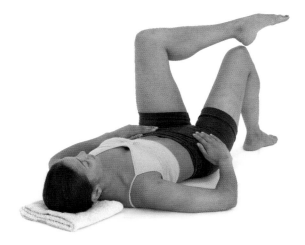

Double Knee Fold

This exercise looks deceptively easy but is, in fact, one of the hardest exercises in the book!

Bringing the knees onto the chest one at a time without allowing the lower abdominals to bulge and without losing neutral requires excellent core stability. We have given you two levels of difficulty. It is easier to learn Double Knee Folds in reverse: that is lowering the feet to the floor rather than lifting them off. It gives you some idea of the strength and control you will need to do Stage 2.

You may need to zip up strongly for a Double Knee Fold, see page 42.

Srarting Position: Stage 1
Lie in the Relaxation Position (page 34).

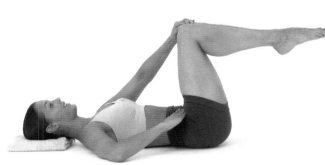

Action

1 Breathe in wide and full to prepare.
2 Breathe out, zip up and hollow and stay zipped throughout. Fold one knee up, staying in neutral and keeping the lower abdominals hollow (as for Knee Folds on page 48).
3 Breathe in and take hold of the raised knee lightly with one or both hands.
4 Breathe out and fold the second knee up so that both knees are now bent at an angle so it looks as though you are sitting on a chair (lying on your back, of course). Line your feet up so the toes are lightly touching; the knees stay hip-width apart.
5 Now for the hard bit: let go of the knee. Breathe in, lengthen through the spine and check that your pelvis is in neutral and your low back feels anchored (using your zip).
6 Breathe out, still zipped, and slowly lower one foot to the floor. Do not allow the abdominals to bulge or lose neutral.
7 Breathe in, then out, and slowly lower the other foot.
8 Repeat 6 times, alternating which leg you raise and lower first.

> **watchpoints**
>
> - You will be surprised at how the body tries to cheat and use everything other than the lower abdominals to stabilize you. Be aware of this and keep your neck and shoulders relaxed.
> - Use the right amount of zip. Zip up slowly and gently to start with and then increase your zip if you need to.
> - Keep your sacrum square on the mat, the tailbone down.
> - Keep the back of your neck long.
> - Your lower abdominals must stay hollow and scooped throughout.

Double Knee Fold Continued

Starting Position: Stage 2

Lie in the Relaxation Position (page 34).

Action

1 Breathe in wide and full to prepare.
2 Breathe out, zip up and hollow and stay zipped throughout. Fold one knee up. The lower abdominals stay
  hollow; the pelvis in neutral.
3 Breathe in wide and full.
4 Breathe out and fold the other knee in. Stay zipped,
  hollowed and neutral.
5 Breathe in wide.
6 Breathe out and lower the first leg you raised.
7 Breathe in then out, and lower the second leg.
8 Repeat 6 times, alternating which leg you raise and
  lower first.

watchpoints
• As for Stage 1.

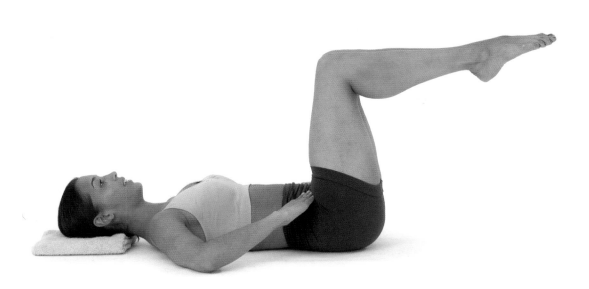

Scapular Stability

The final part of our girdle of strength concerns the muscles of the mid back, those which set the shoulder blades down into the back. They are the lower trapezius and the serratus anterior muscles. When they are working correctly they stabilize the scapulae, placing them and the shoulder joints in the best position to allow for good mechanics. By strengthening these muscles you are also helping to prevent those unsightly flaps of flabby skin which can hang like curtains from your shoulder blades!

These exercises are designed to open out the chest, teach good alignment of the head, neck and shoulders, and strengthen the stabilizing muscles. The idea is to re-educate your movement so when you reach up with your arms the action is free-flowing and natural.

To find these muscles, try the following exercises.

Shoulder Reach 1

The goal of these two exercises is to be aware of the muscles in the mid back that connect the shoulder blades down into the back.

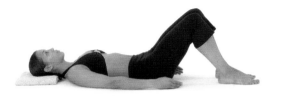

Starting Position for 1 and 2

Lie in the Relaxation Position (page 34). Have your arms resting down by your sides, palms facing inwards. Go through your relaxation checklist.

Action

1 Breathe in wide to prepare and lengthen through the spine.

2 Breathe out, zip up and hollow, and slide your arms down towards your feet, reaching through the fingertips and turning your palms to face inwards. As you do so you will feel your shoulder blades connecting down into your back and your upper-body will open out.

3 Breathe in and hold the stretch; be aware of the distance between your ears and your shoulders.

4 Breathe out and relax.

5 Repeat 5 times.

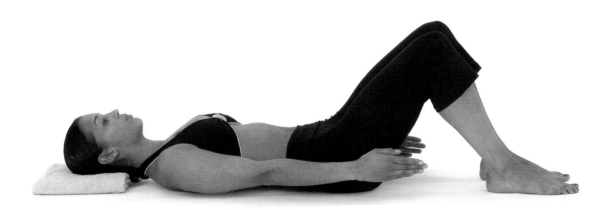

Shoulder Reach 2

Action

1 Follow actions 1 and 2 for Shoulder Reach 1. Then, on the same out-breath raise both arms so they are directly above your shoulders.
2 Keep your shoulder blades down into the mat.
3 Breathe in and return to the starting position.
4 Repeat 5 times.

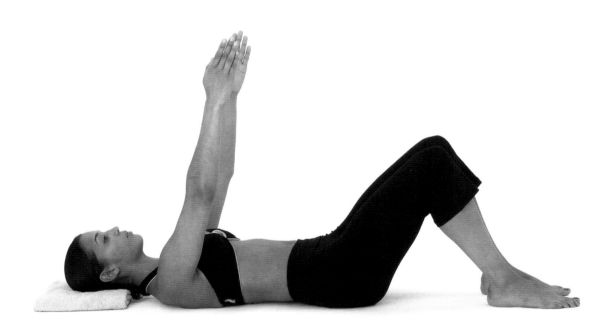

Dart Stage 1

We are now going to find the same muscles, but this time we will do so lying face down.

Equipment

A flat pillow (optional).

Starting Position

Lie face down (if you prefer, you can place a flat pillow under your forehead to allow you to breathe) with your arms by your sides and palms facing the ceiling. Your neck is long, your legs relaxed and together in parallel.

Action

1 Breathe in to prepare and lengthen through the spine, tucking your chin in gently as if you were holding a ripe peach beneath it.
2 Breathe out, zip up and hollow, and slide your shoulder blades down into your back. Turn your palms towards your body, lengthening your fingers down towards your feet.
3 The top of your head stays lengthening away from you too.
4 Keep looking straight down at the floor. Do not tip your head back.
5 Breathe in and feel the length of the body from the tips of your toes to the top of your head.
6 Breathe out, still zipping, and release.

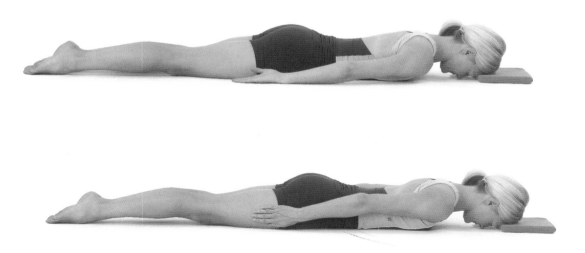

Dart Stage 2

Starting Position

As for Stage 1.

Action

1 Breathe in to prepare and lengthen through the spine. Tuck your chin in gently.

2 Breathe out, zip up and hollow and stay zipped throughout. Slide your shoulder blades down into your back. Turn your palms towards your body and lengthen your fingers away from you down towards your feet. Keep looking straight down at the floor. Squeeze your inner thighs together but keep your feet on the floor. At the same time, slowly lift your upper body from the floor. Don't come up too high, just a few inches. Use your mid, not lower, back muscles.

3 Breathe in and feel the length of the body from the tips of your toes to the top of your head.

4 Breathe out, still zipping, and lengthen and lower back down.

5 Repeat 6 times, then move into the Rest Position (page 58).

---

watchpoints stages 1 and 2

- Keep zipping throughout.
- Keep your focus down.
- Do not strain the neck; it should feel released as your shoulders engage down into your back. Think of a swan's neck growing out between its wings.
- Remember to keep your feet on the floor.
- Stop if you feel at all uncomfortable in the low back. This exercise can also be done with the feet hip-width apart and the thigh and buttock muscles relaxed.

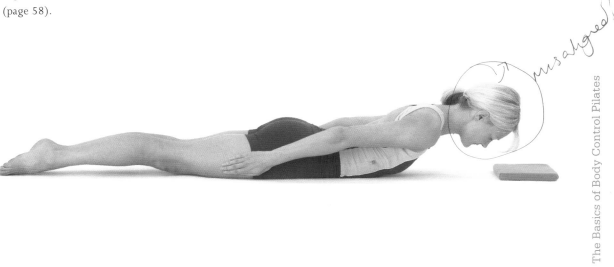

misaligned?

Rest Position

This is a lovely way to stretch out the back especially after doing any exercise in which you are lying on your front or are in four-point kneeling.

Equipment

A plump cushion (optional).

Starting Position

Come onto all fours. Have your hands directly beneath your shoulders, your knees beneath your hips. Your spine should be long, retaining its natural curves. Look down at the floor to keep the back of your neck long. Your legs should be in parallel. Keep your elbows soft and your shoulder blades down into your back.

> Avoid the Rest Position if you have knee problems because you can compress the joint. You may like to put a cushion under the knees to reduce the pressure on the joints.

Action

1 Bring your feet together, keeping your knees apart. Slowly move back towards your buttocks. Do not raise your head or hands and come back to sit on your feet, not between them. The back is rounded. Rest and relax into this position. Leave the arms extended to give you the maximum stretch. Feel the expansion of the back of your ribcage as you breathe deeply into it.

2 The further apart the knees are, the more of a stretch you will feel in your inner thighs.

3 With the knees further apart, you can really think of your chest sinking down into the floor.

4 Take up to 10 breaths in this position.

To Come Out of Rest Position

As you breathe out, zip up and hollow and slowly unfurl. Think of dropping your tailbone down and bringing your pubic bone forwards. Rebuild your spine vertebra by vertebra until you are upright.

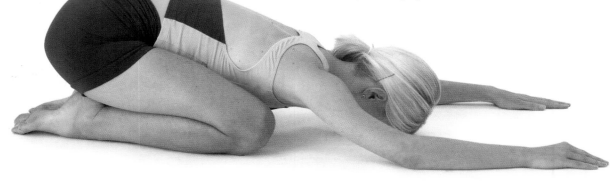

watchpoints

- Use cushions wherever you need them!
- Really try to breathe deeply into your low back.
- Always come back up slowly and with control, bone by bone, bringing your head up last.

Neck Rolls and Chin Tucks

This basic skill will help you position your head on your neck correctly, releasing tension and mobilizing the spine. You use this 'nod' when you perform many of the exercises in the main programme. Think about the lovely long graceful neck of a dancer. This exercise will help you achieve a similar look.

An important aspect of re-educating the head–neck relationship lies in the relative strength of the neck extensors (which tilt the head back) and flexors (which tilt the head forward). If you think about the body positioned at a desk or steering wheel, the head is usually thrust forward and tipped back creating a muscle imbalance. By relaxing the jaw, lengthening the back of the neck and gently tucking the chin in, this balance can be redressed.

Starting Position

Lie in the Relaxation Position (page 34) with your knees bent and your arms resting on your lower abdomen. Only use a flat pillow if you are uncomfortable without one; your head will roll better if you do not use one.

Action

1 Release your neck and jaw, allowing your tongue to widen at its base. Keep the neck nicely lengthened and soften your breastbone. Allow the shoulder blades to widen and melt into the floor.
2 Now, allow your head to roll slowly to one side.
3 Bring it back to the centre and over to the other side, taking your time.
4 When the neck feels free, bring the head to the centre and gently tuck your chin in, as if holding a ripe peach under it (you do not want to crush the delicate skin). Keep the head on the floor and lengthen out of the back of the neck.
5 Return the head to the centre.
6 Repeat the rolling to the side and chin tuck 8 times.

This is a subtle movement – you should tuck your chin in gently. It is a nodding action.

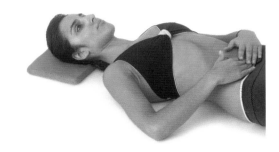

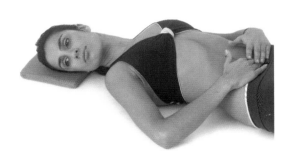

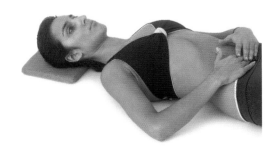

watchpoints

- Do not force the head or neck, just let it roll naturally.
- Do not lift the head off the floor when you tuck the chin in.

Floating Arms

With good movement, the shoulder blade will move in the same way as the ballast on a security barrier would move.

We all have a tendency to overuse the upper part of our shoulders (the upper trapezius). As you raise your arm in the exercise think of this order of movement:

- First, just your arm moves up and out.
- Then, you will feel the shoulder blade start to move as it coils down and around the back of the ribcage and under towards the armpit.
- Finally, the collar bone (clavicle) will rise up.

Starting Position

Stand tall. Place your left hand on your right shoulder, so you can feel your collar bone. You are going to try to keep it still for the first part of the movement. Your hand checks that the upper part of your shoulder remains 'quiet' for as long as possible. Very often this part will overwork, so think of it staying soft and released, while the lower trapezius below your shoulder blades works to set the shoulder blades down into your back.

Action

1 Breathe in to prepare and lengthen up through the spine, letting the neck relax.
2 Breathe out and zip up and hollow. Slowly begin to raise the arm, reaching wide out of the shoulder blades like a bird's wing. Think of the hand as leading the arm, the arm following the hand as it floats upwards.
3 Rotate the arm so that the palm opens to the ceiling as the arm reaches shoulder level. Try to keep the shoulder under your hand as still as possible and the shoulder blade dropping down into your back for as long as possible.
4 Breathe in as you lower the arm to your side.
5 Repeat 3 times with each arm.

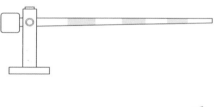

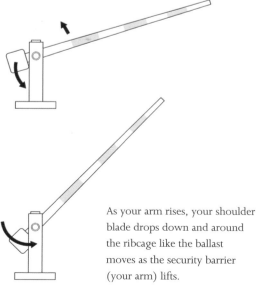

As your arm rises, your shoulder blade drops down and around the ribcage like the ballast moves as the security barrier (your arm) lifts.

---

watchpoints

- Keep a sense of openness in the upper body.
- Do not allow your upper body to shift to the side, keep centred.
- Keep your ribs calm and down; do not allow them to flare.
- Do not lean backwards.

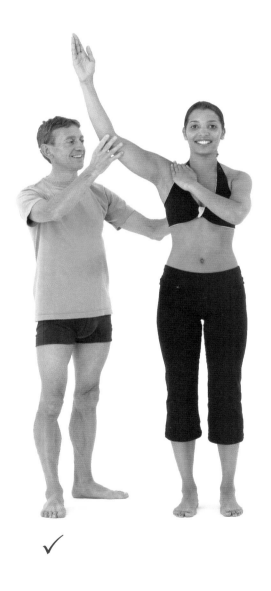

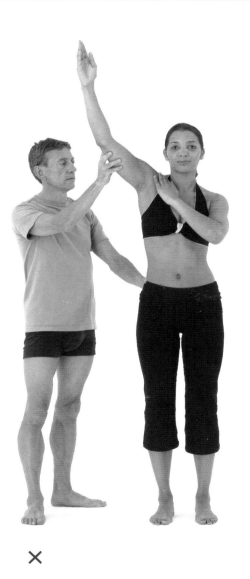

✓

✗

Starfish – Arms Only

As your arm moves back think of what you learnt in Floating Arms (page 60). Focus on keeping the upper shoulders relaxed and the ribcage down. You can also do this exercise with the palms facing inwards. This is particularly recommended if you have a shoulder problem.

Starting Position

Lie in the Relaxation Position (page 34) with your arms down by your sides.

Action

1 Breathe wide into your lower ribcage to prepare.
2 Breathe out, zip up and hollow, and start to take one arm back as if to touch the floor. You may not be able to do this comfortably, so only move the arm as far as you are happy to do so.
3 Do not force the arm, keep it soft and open with the elbow bent. Think of the shoulder blade setting down into your back. The ribs stay calm. Do not allow the back to arch at all.
4 Breathe in, still zipped, as you return the arm to your side.
5 Repeat 5 times with each arm.

watchpoints

- Do not take the arm too close to your head.
- Keep the elbow bent a little.

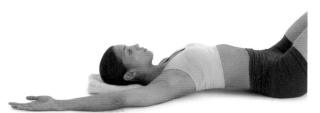

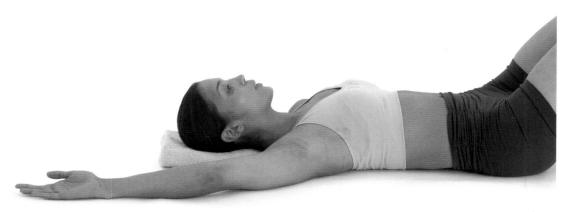

Full Starfish

Now you are going to co-ordinate the opposite arm and leg movement, away from your strong centre. Although this looks simple, it is a sophisticated movement pattern, using all the skills of good movement learnt so far. This may also be done with the palms facing the body. This is particular recommended if you have a shoulder problem.

Starting Position

Lie in the Relaxation Position (page 34), with your arms down by your sides.

Action

1 Breathe in wide and full to prepare.
2 Breathe out, zip up and hollow. Slide the left leg away along the floor in a line with your hips and take the right arm above you in a backstroke movement. Keep the pelvis completely neutral, stable and still, and the stomach muscles engaged. Keep the ribcage down, and a sense of width and openness in the upper body and shoulders.
3 Breathe in, still zipped and hollowed, and return the limbs to the starting position.
4 Repeat 5 times alternating arms and legs.

watchpoints

- Do not be tempted to over-reach; the 'girdle of strength' must stay in place.
- Slide the leg in a line with the hip.
- Make sure the ribcage stays down.

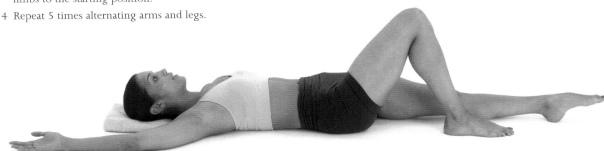

Basic Curl Up

The perfect curl up is one of the secrets to achieving a flat stomach. Do not be tempted to rush this exercise – slow, controlled, precise movement gets results!

Starting Position

Lie in the Relaxation Position (page 34). Gently release your neck by rolling the head slowly from side to side. Lightly clasp your hands behind your head to cradle and support the head (at no point should you pull on your neck). Keep your elbows open just in front of your ears throughout.

Action

1 Breathe in, wide and full, to prepare.
2 Breathe out and zip up and hollow. Soften your breast-bone, tuck your chin in a little (as if holding a ripe peach) and curl up, breaking from the breastbone. Your stomach must not pop up. Keep the pelvis level and the tailbone down on the floor lengthening away.
3 Breathe in and slowly curl back down, controlling the movement.
4 Repeat 10 times.

Avoid this exercise if you have neck problems.

watchpoints

- Try not to grip around the hips, keep the muscles soft.
- Stay in neutral, tailbone down on the floor and lengthening away. The front of the body keeps its length, A useful image is that there is a strip of sticky tape along the front of the body which should not wrinkle!
- Think of peeling the upper spine bone by bone from the floor.
- Think of the ribs funnelling down towards the waist.
- Keep the chin gently tucked in. This is the cervical nod action you learnt in Neck Rolls and Chin Tucks on page 59, which should help keep your neck released.
- Don't close your elbows as you come up, keep them open but within your peripheral vision.

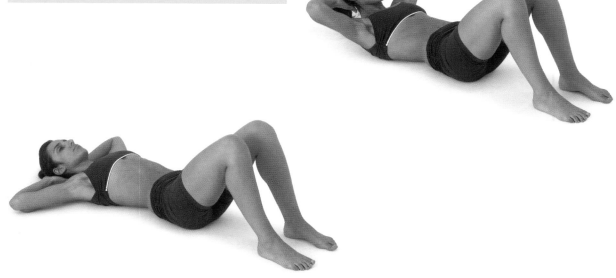

We have grouped the exercises according to which parts of the body they work on most: abdominals, bottom, legs, shoulders, etc. This will give you an idea of which exercises are of greatest value to your body shape. However, you should bear in mind that Pilates exercises always affect the whole body, even the non-moving parts! For example, in Side Kick Variation on page 90 you are working the deep muscles which hold the trunk still while the legs move. This is why Pilates is a total body conditioning method.

The exercises are not in any set order; for balanced workouts please turn to page 123.

The Exercises

The photograph on page 2 should be enough to convince you just how awful bad posture looks. The quickest way to look like you have lost 2.5 kilos (5 pounds) is to stop slouching and stand up tall.

The following exercises have been chosen because they work on your awareness of what good posture is and also strengthen the muscles you need to maintain it 24/7.

This series of exercises challenges your sense of balance and your proprioception (that is your body's awareness of its position in space). Once you have tried them a few times you can add the different foot positions to some of your standing Pilates exercises, such as Cleopatra on page 72. These exercises will also help prepare you for the Upright Chair Stretch on page 92.

The idea is progressively to narrow your base of support by changing the foot position/coming onto one foot and then adding the challenge of removing your visual input.

Clear the furniture for this one in case your proprioception fails you!

The action is the same for each position. Notice how your body compensates with each change.

Position 1: Standing Well

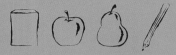

Position 2: Standing with Feet Together

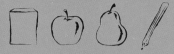

Stand correctly, following the directions below.

Starting Position

Stand correctly, following the directions below, but this time have your feet together in parallel. Line up the joints. Engage your inner thighs and gently lift your buttock muscles.

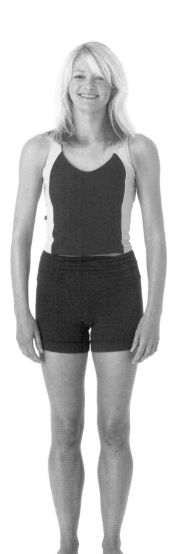

- Allow your head to go forward and up.

- Allow your neck to release.

- Keep your breastbone soft.

- Keep your shoulder blades down into your back.

- Lengthen up through the spine.

- Your elbows are open.

- Check your pelvis: is it in neutral?

- Gently zip up and hollow.

- Release your knees so they are not locked back.

- Keep the weight even on both feet; do not allow them to roll in or out. Think of three points; base of the big toes, base of the small toes, centre of the heels.

- Your feet should be hip-width apart in parallel or with a slight natural turn-out if more comfortable.

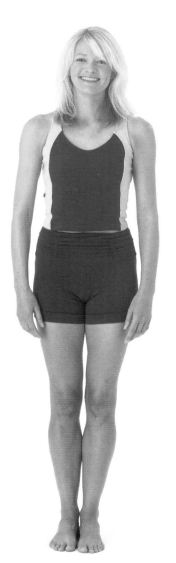

Position 3: Pilates Stance

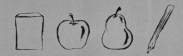

This traditional Pilates Stance helps tone the buttocks and the inner thighs.

Starting Position

Stand tall with your legs and feet naturally turned out, but with the heels touching and the legs together. Follow the directions given for Standing Well, but this time engage your inner thighs and also the deep muscles which 'wrap around' deep in your buttocks.

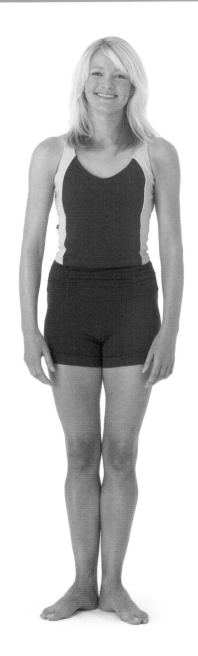

Position 4:
Standing on One Leg

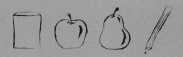

Starting Position

Stand on one foot. You can experiment with having the foot hip-width (in a line with the centre of your buttock) or central. Rest the foot of the non-supporting leg on the inside of the opposite calf. You will naturally transfer your weight, but your pelvis should remain level. This is quite difficult and you must remember to zip. You can also try engaging the working buttock by gently sucking it in (as if you are sucking in your cheeks).

Action for Positions 1–4

1 Close one eye; be aware of how this feels. Open the eye.
2 Repeat with the other eye.
3 Close both eyes.
4 Then, for Position 4, reverse the feet.

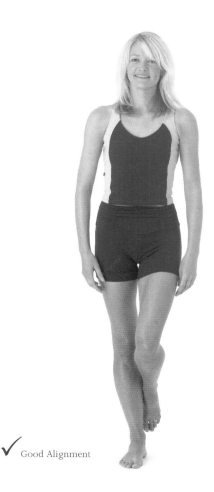

✓ Good Alignment

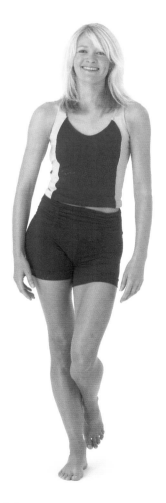

✗ Incorrect: the pelvis is not level.

Standing Hundred – Breathing Versions 1–3

This useful standing exercise gives you a deep abdominal workout, tones the arms and shoulder area and gets your blood pumping. It's a great way to wake up, energize your body and focus the mind. It teaches you to co-ordinate breathing with movement.

You will use this same breathing pattern when you do Circles Adduction on page 88.

Equipment

Stretch band or scarf (optional).

Starting Position for Versions 1 and 2

Stand tall, remembering all the directions from Standing Well on page 67. Either put your hands on your ribcage or wrap a scarf or stretch band around it.

Action for Version 1

1 Breathe in and feel the ribcage expand.
2 Breathe out, zip up and hollow and stay zipped throughout.
3 Breathe in to a count of 3 and feel the ribs expanding.
4 Breathe out to a count of 3 and feel the ribs close down.
5 Repeat up to 10 times.

Action for Version 2

As above, but breathe in and out to a count of 5.

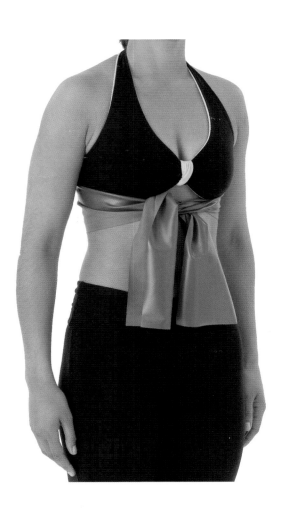
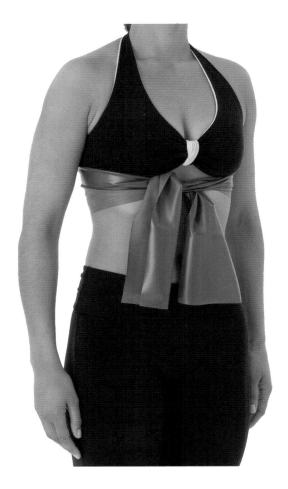

Starting Position for Version 3

We are now ready to add the arm action, so stand tall and stretch your arms down by your sides. Have your palms facing back. Reach through the fingertips and connect your shoulder blades down into your back.

watchpoints

- The arms move from the shoulder joint; the trunk stays still.
- Keep your upper body open.
- Maintain the distance between the ears and the shoulders.
- Keep reaching away through the fingertips.
- Release your neck.
- Keep your wrists strong; don't flap your hands.

Action

1 Breathe in wide to a count of 5. Lengthen up through the spine.
2 Breathe out for a count of 5, zip up and hollow and stay zipped throughout.
3 Continue with this pattern of breathing while pumping the arms back and forth about 15 cm (6 in) in front of and behind the body. Do 5 beats on the in-breath and 5 beats on the out-breath.
4 Repeat until you have counted up to 100 beats of the arms.

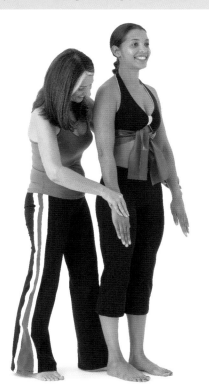

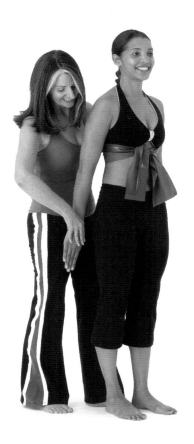

Cleopatra

The aim is to work the arms and upper body and also to teach good upper-body posture. To become aware of the shoulder blades and their relationship with the ribcage and the movement of the arms. To open the chest, especially the muscles at the front of the upper arms/shoulders.

At first glance there seems to be a lot of breathing during this exercise. Use the breath to control your movements and help you focus your mind on which muscles are working around the shoulder girdle.

Starting Position

Stand tall remembering the directions on page 67. Bend your arms to 90 degrees with the palms facing upwards and the tips of your fingers pointing in front of you. Have your elbows tucked into your waist.

Action

1 Breathe in to prepare and lengthen up through the spine.
2 Breathe out, zip up and hollow and stay zipped throughout.
3 Breathe in and, keeping your elbows into your sides, take your hands outwards and back, opening them as far as is comfortable. The movement comes from the shoulder joint.

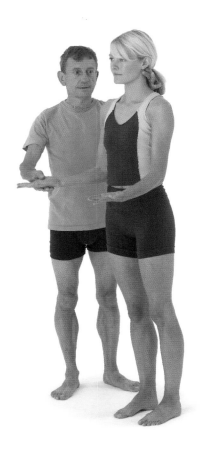
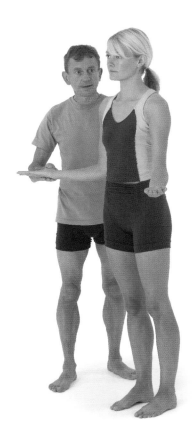

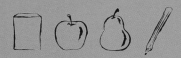

To strengthen the muscles between the shoulder blades.
All this is to be done with the shoulder blades set down into
the back, stabilized.

4 Breathe out and extend the arms out to the sides so they are at shoulder height.
5 Breathe in and turn the palms downwards – only the arms move – the movement originates from the shoulder joint. Keep your upper shoulders relaxed and maintain the distance between ears and shoulders.

6 Breathe out and turn the palms up again, rotating the arms from the shoulders. Keep your shoulder blades down into your back.
7 Breathe in and bend the arms back so the elbows are into the waist.
8 Breathe out and bring the hands back to the starting position.
9 Repeat 4 times.

watchpoints

- Do not allow the upper back to arch as you take the arms back.
- Keep your neck released.
- Keep your arms in your peripheral vision.

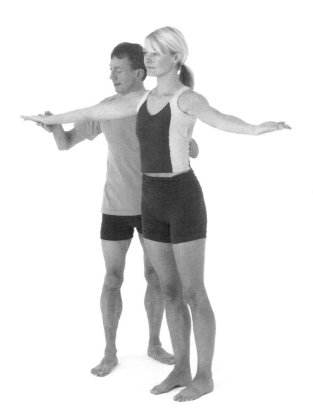

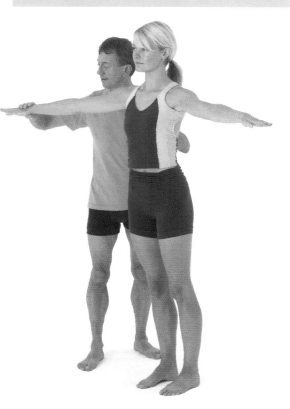

Standing Arm Openings

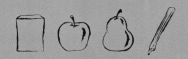

A gentle, feel-good exercise that opens the upper body, rotating the spine and working the shoulders and waist muscles.

Starting Position

Stand in the Pilates Stance (page 68). Have your arms out in front of you at shoulder height as if hugging a large tree. Shoulders are down. Neck is released. Elbows are facing outwards.

watchpoints

- Keep your peripheral focus on your fingers.
- Remember your pelvis stays still, facing front.
- Soften between your shoulder blades as you turn.
- Float the arm around.
- Keep lengthening through the middle finger.
- Maintain distance between ears and shoulders.

Action

1 Breathe in wide and lengthen up through the spine.
2 Breathe out, zip up and hollow and stay zipped throughout. Keep the right arm still and start to rotate your trunk to the left, taking the left arm with you. Your head follows the movement. Your pelvis stays put! Only open the arm as far as is comfortable.
3 Breathe in and return.
4 Repeat 3 times on each side, alternating.
5 You could also turn on the in-breath.
6 You can vary the standing position (see pages 67–9).

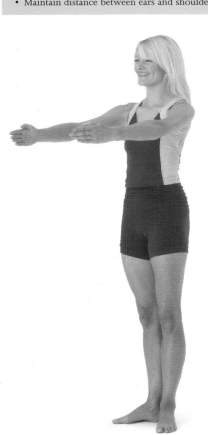

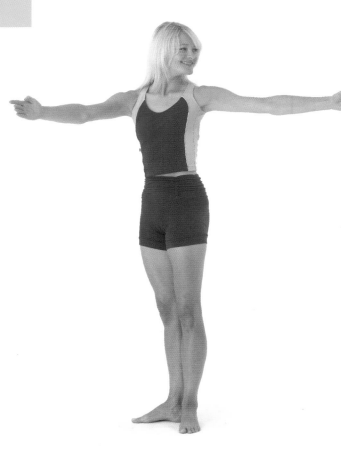

Few women are happy with their lower halves! Notoriously hard to tone, we promise that these exercises will reach the parts other techniques have failed to reach. They are perfect for achieving sculpted, firm and shapely bottoms, thighs and calves. They will even help reduce cellulite.

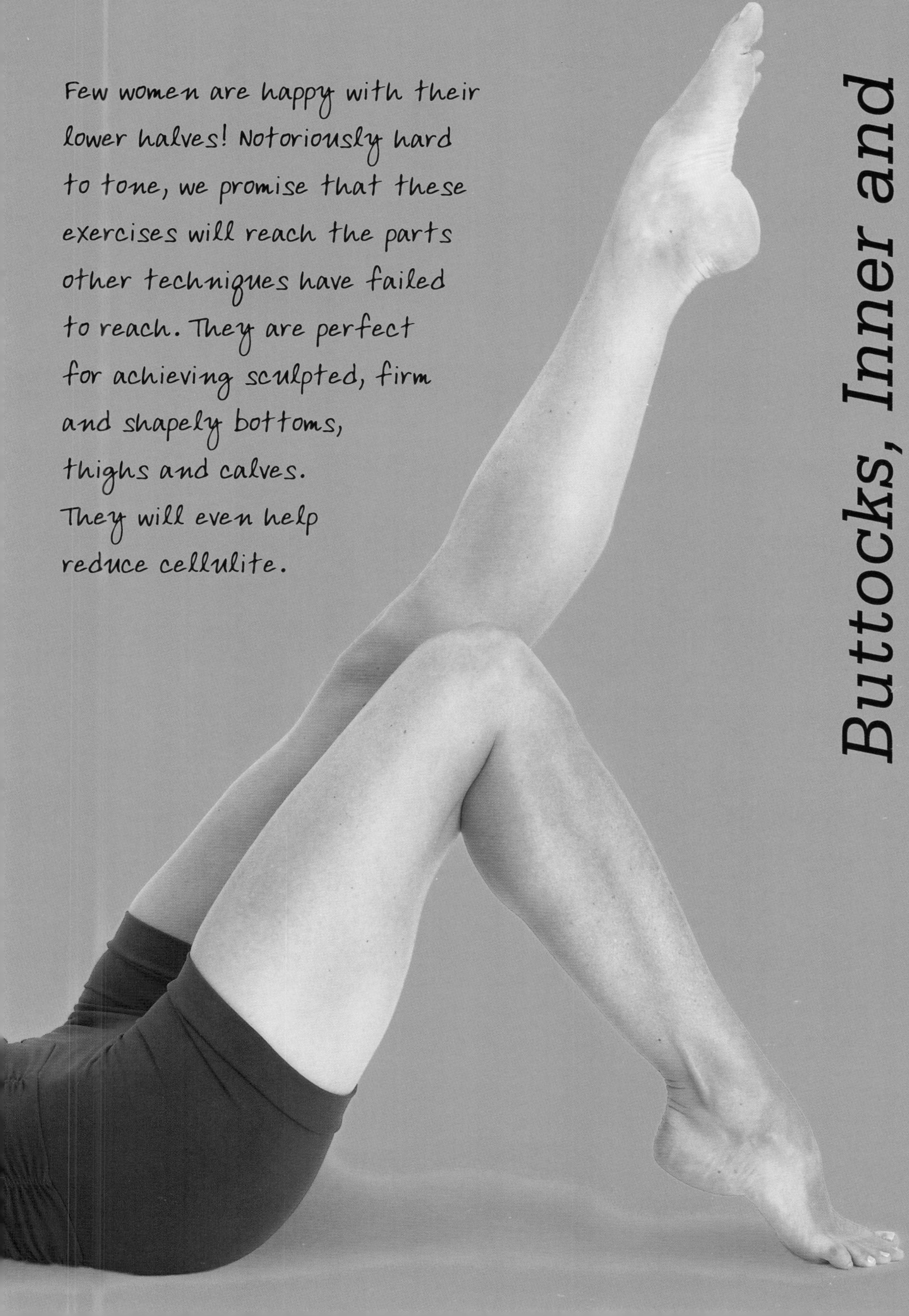

Buttocks, Inner and Outer Thighs and Calves

Leg Shaper

This exercise is incredibly effective at sculpting the legs. It can be done with or without the use of a step. The step provides a calf stretch, but the exercise works well without it.

Equipment

Two tennis balls, or one tennis ball and a small cushion.

Starting Position

Stand tall with the feet hip-width apart and in parallel. If you are using a step, you will need to hold the banister. For safety, the bottom step is best. Have the balls of your feet firmly planted on the step, the arches and the heels over the edge. If you don't have a step you won't get the calf stretch, but you can still work the legs and if you don't hold on you can also work on your balance. Put one tennis ball between your ankles just beneath the ankle bones. The other tennis ball (or you could use a very small cushion) goes between your legs just above the knees. The idea is that the balls keep your legs in good alignment.

Action

1 Breathe normally throughout and remain gently zipped.
2 Bend both knees directly over your second toes, maintain good posture, do not tip forwards or backwards.

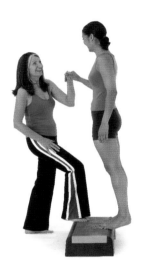

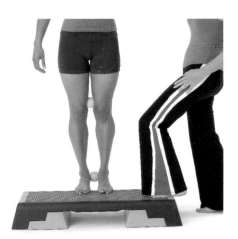

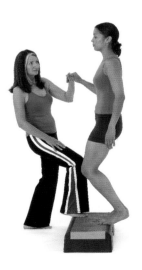

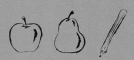

3 Lift both heels so you are on the balls of your feet. Knees are still bent. Keep lengthening upwards. Don't stick your bottom out!

4 Slowly straighten your legs but stay on the balls of your feet.

5 Now lower your heels away from the top of your head until, if you are on a flat surface, they reach the floor or, if you are on a step, they lower over the edge to stretch your calves.

6 Repeat 10 times.

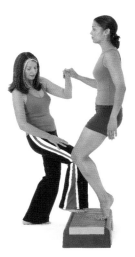

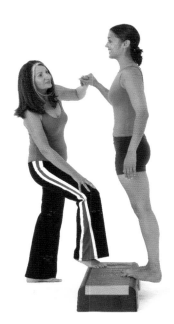

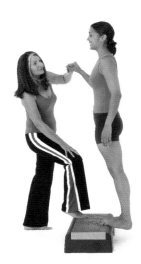

The Exercises

Leg Sweeps

This exercise is a choreographed sequence of pelvic stability exercises. It will strengthen your abdomen, hips and thighs, and tests and challenges your core stability. Try to keep the movement smooth and flowing. Move with awareness and control.

Starting Position

Adopt the Relaxation Position (page 34). Check your pelvis is in neutral, your tailbone down and lengthening away. Keep your hands on your pelvic bones to check for unwanted movement.

Action

1 Breathe in wide and full to prepare.
2 Breathe out, zip up and hollow and stay zipped throughout. Slide one leg away along the floor, keeping the lower abdominals engaged and the pelvis still, stable and in neutral.
3 Breathe in and flex the foot, lengthening away through the heel.
4 As you breathe out, sweep the leg up, lifting from underneath but keeping your tailbone down and your pelvis level.
5 Breathe in again, relax the foot and bend the knee in. Keep the pelvis still and the tailbone down.
6 Breathe out and replace the foot on the floor, ready to start again.
7 Repeat 5 times with the same leg before changing legs.

watchpoints

- Remember you are trying to avoid even the slightest movement of the pelvis.
- It helps to think of the waist being long and even on both sides as you make the movement.
- Remember to keep your pelvic floor engaged and your lower abdominals hollowed throughout.
- As you sweep the leg up, keep it in a line with your hips. Try not to overuse the quadriceps muscles at the front of your thighs. Use your core.
- Try to keep your neck and jaw released throughout.

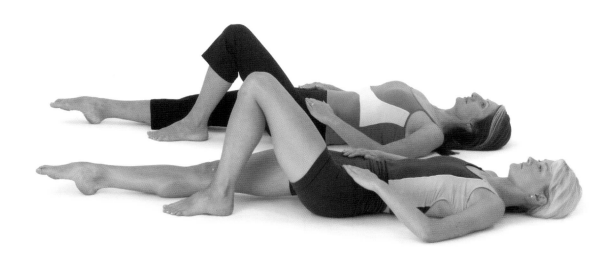

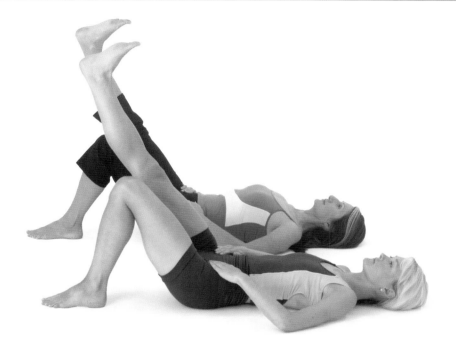

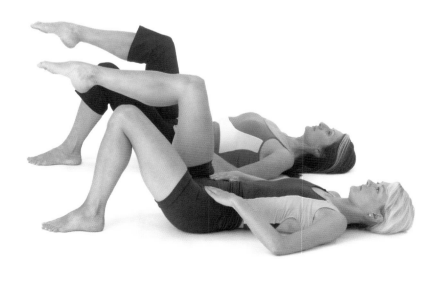

Spine Curls with Arm Circles

Another fun combination exercise. This one tones your bottom, abdomen, arms and shoulders. You use your deep buttock muscles to stay in the bridge position, which helps promote pelvic stability and develops segmental control of the spine and good scapulo-humeral rhythm.

Starting Position

Lie in the Relaxation Position (page 34) with your feet about 20 cm (8 in) from your buttocks, hip-width apart and parallel. Plant the feet firmly into the floor. Your arms rest down by your sides. Reach through the fingertips. Keep the shoulder blades connected down into the back.

Action for Arm Circles

1 Breathe in wide and full. Lengthen through the body.
2 Breathe out, zip up and hollow and stay zipped throughout. Raise your arms up and take them behind you. Palms facing up.
3 Breathe in as you circle the arms out to the sides and back down to your body; turn the palms down as you reach your body. Keep your arms 7–8 cm (3–4 in) off the floor.
4 Repeat 5 times, then reverse the direction of the circle and repeat another 5 times.

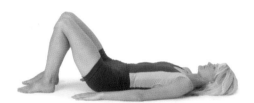

watchpoints
• Maintain neutral pelvis and neutral spine throughout and do not allow the upper back to arch.
• Do not allow the ribs to flare. Move with the breath.
• Keep the shoulder blades wide and down the back, but do allow for mobility. No gripping!
• Keep the neck long and released.
• Watch the alignment of the hands and wrists.
• Keep the elbows soft.

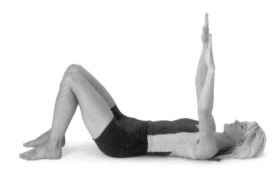

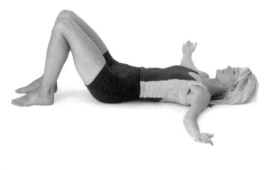

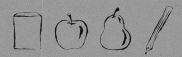

We have broken the exercises down, so as a preparation you practise the arm circles before you add them to the spine curl. Once you are confident that your arm circles are proficient try the full version.

Action for Spine Curls

1 Breathe in wide and full to prepare.
2 Breathe out, zip up and hollow and stay zipped throughout. Engage your buttock muscles and curl your tailbone off the mat. You will lose the neutral pelvis position.
3 Breathe in, then out and roll back down to neutral.
4 Repeat 5 times, lifting a little more of the spine off the floor each time. Move the spine in sequence, bone by bone. Breathe out as you move the spine.

Action for Spine Curls with Arm Circles

1 Breathe in. As you breathe out, zip up and hollow and wheel the spine up bone by bone from the mat. Do not go higher than the shoulder blades.
2 Breathe in. As you breathe out, raise your arms and circle them above your head. Keep your arms a few centimetres off the floor. Keep your ribcage closed down.
3 Breathe in as you circle your arms around and back down to your sides, turning the palms down as you go.
4 Breathe out and wheel the spine back down.
5 Repeat 3 times.

When you are proficient at this exercise you can use light hand weights of 0.5 kg (1 lb) each to build tone in your arms.

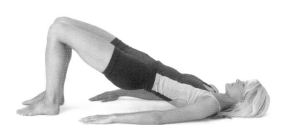

watchpoints	

- Take care your back does not arch as your arms circle!
- Do not rush the first few Spine Curls. Really make the base of the spine move.
- Do not allow your feet to roll in or out. Keep them grounded.
- Do not allow the ribs to flare.
- Keep the shoulder blades wide and down the back, but do allow for mobility, no gripping!
- Keep the neck long and released.
- Watch the alignment of the hands and wrists.
- Keep the elbows soft.

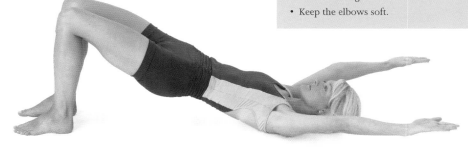

The Exercises

Bottom Worker

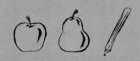

You can actually feel your bottom tightening as you do this exercise! You will feel your gluteals working harder with each bounce, and it will mobilize the lower vertebrae.

Equipment

A small cushion. A flat pillow or folded towel (optional). You will need to clear a space on a wall.

Starting Position

Most mats will move too much, so unless you have a non-slip one it is better just to lie directly on the floor. Lie by a wall with your knees bent at right angles and your feet together on the wall. Place a small cushion between your knees. If you are very round-shouldered, you may need a flat pillow or folded towel under your head. Have your arms down by your sides.

> This is a challenging exercise; approach it with caution and stop if it causes discomfort.
> Do not do it if you have low back problems.

Action

1 Breathe in and lengthen through the spine.
2 Breathe out, zip up and hollow and stay zipped throughout. Gently squeeze the cushion and your buttocks, and slowly curl your spine bone by bone from the floor as far as the bottom of your shoulder blades. Hold this position.
3 Breathing normally, continue to squeeze the cushion and your buttocks as you gently bounce up and down. It's a small movement. Keep squeezing and zipping.
4 You are aiming for 20 bounces, but stop when you need to.
5 On an out-breath replace the spine on the floor slowly bone by bone.
6 Repeat up to 3 times.

watchpoints

- Keep the back of your neck long.
- Keep reaching through your fingertips; slide the shoulder blades down constantly.
- Keep breathing!
- Keep squeezing that cushion!

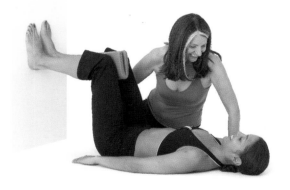

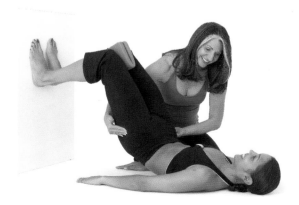

Star Test

This is a core Body Control exercise. This simple version really helps you to isolate the right muscles - in this case the buttocks - while maintaining good alignment.

Equipment

A flat pillow or folded towel.

It is useful to lie on a very thin mat or even the floor for this exercise because you get better feedback.

Starting Position

Lie on your front in a straight line. Put a flat pillow or folded towel under your forehead. Place your fingertips underneath your hips. The idea is that you keep your hip bones still. If your pelvis tilts, you will feel it. In fact, you will squash your fingers!

Action

1 Breathe in wide and full and lengthen through the spine.
2 Breathe out, zip up and hollow, and lengthen and lift your right leg a few centimetres from the floor. There should be no extra pressure on your fingertips.
3 Breathe in, still zipped, and lengthen and lower the leg.
4 Repeat 6 times with each leg.

watchpoints	

- If it is more comfortable, you can turn your head to one side.
- Keep zipping and hollowing.
- The buttocks and the hamstrings work as you lift the leg. Try to engage the buttocks before the hamstrings.
- Reach out of the hip joint. Keep both hips on the mat!
- Keep the pelvis completely still. Try not to allow it to tip forwards or to one side. You will feel the change in pressure on your fingertips if this happens.
- Your upper body should remain relaxed but not collapsed; keep your shoulder blades down into your back and your neck released.

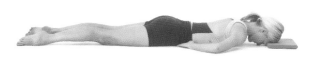

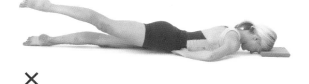

✗

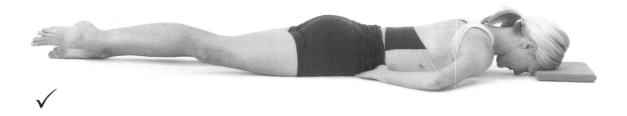

✓

Oyster 1 and 2

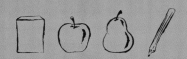

Oyster and Charleston are great exercises to mobilize your hip joints and trim your buttocks and waist muscles. The action of turning out the leg is an excellent preparation for the more classical Side Kick Variation on page 90.

Do Oyster 1 and 2 and Charleston in turn on one side, then turn over and repeat them on the other side.

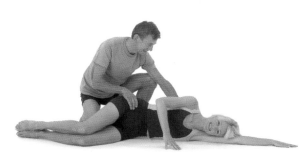

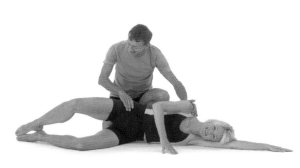

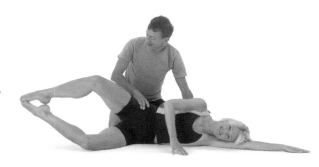

Equipment
A small flat pillow or a folded towel (optional).

Starting Position for Oyster and Charleston
Lie on your side in a straight line. Use the edge of your mat as a guide. Your underneath arm is stretched out in line with your body. You can put a pillow between your ear and arm so your neck keeps in line with your spine. Bend your knees, keeping the soles of your feet in line with your bottom. Line your joints up: ankle over ankle; knee over knee; shoulder over shoulder. Your hips stay square; your waist is lifted.

Action for Oyster 1
1 Breathe in wide and full to prepare.
2 Breathe out, zip up and hollow and stay zipped throughout. Slowly rotate your top leg, opening the knee. Keep your lower foot on the floor. Both feet touch each other. Do not move your trunk at all; your pelvis stays still. The action originates deep in the buttocks.
3 Breathe in and hold the position.
4 Breathe out and slowly close the knees.
5 Repeat 5 times.

Action for Oyster 2
1 Breathe in wide and full to prepare.
2 Breathe out, zip up and hollow and stay zipped throughout. Slowly rotate your top leg, opening the knee and simultaneously lifting both feet from the floor. Keep the feet glued together. The thigh of your bottom leg stays down. Do not fall forwards or backwards. Your waist stays lifted.
3 Breathe in and hold the position.
4 Breathe out, lower and close.
5 Repeat 5 times.

Charleston

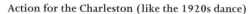

Action for the Charleston (like the 1920s dance)

1 Breathe in wide and full to prepare.
2 Breathe out, zip up and hollow and stay zipped throughout.
3 Breathe in and, keeping the knees together, lift the top foot. The ankle in the air stays over the ankle below. The movement comes from the hip joint. The pelvis stays still and square.
4 Breathe out and return to the starting position.
5 Repeat 5 times.

watchpoints for Oyster 1 and 2 and Charleston

- Do not allow the waist to sink into the floor; keep it long and lifted.
- Do not allow upper body to collapse forward.
- Keep the neck long and your focus forward.
- Maintain a neutral pelvis throughout.
- Be aware of your feet.

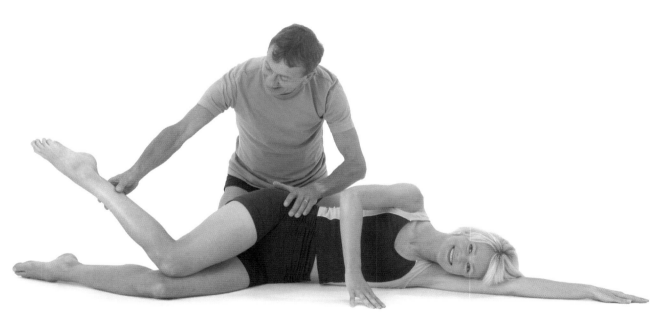

Boxes Abduction

This and the following exercise, challenge and tone your hips and outer and inner thighs, helping to prevent cellulite. They also work your abdominals and waist muscles because you have to hold your trunk still while the legs move.

Equipment

Practise these exercises first without weights, until you are totally familiar and comfortable with them. You can then strap leg weights of 1–1.5 kg (2.5–3 lb) each on to your ankles. Start with the lightest weight.

A small flat pillow or a folded towel (optional).

Starting Position

Lie on your left side in a straight line, shoulder over shoulder, hip over hip, ankle over ankle. Remember neutral spine and pelvis, please. Your left arm is stretched out, your head rests on your arm. You may place a flat pillow between your ear and your arm to fill the gap if you wish. Bring your legs forward until they are at an angle of about 45 degrees to the body. Place your right hand on the floor in front of your chest, with the elbow bent to support you. Throughout the exercise, keep lifting the waist off the floor and maintain the length in the trunk.

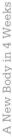

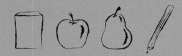

Action

The aim is to draw a rectangular box with your leg, 25 x 15 cm (10 x 6 in).

1 Breathe in wide, breathe out and zip up and hollow and stay zipped throughout. Straighten your top leg, so it is in a line with your hip and about 12 cm (5 in) off the floor. Be careful not to take it behind you! The pelvis stays still, the foot is pointed. Both knees face forward.

2 On your next breath out, slowly bring the leg in front of you about 25 cm (10 in).

3 Breathe in and lift the leg about 15 cm (6 in).

4 Breathe out and bring the leg back 25 cm (10 in) to be in a line with your body.

5 Breathe in and lower the leg 15 cm (6 in) to be in a line with your hip again.

6 Do this, then Circles Adduction, 5 times on one side before rolling onto the other side and repeating them 5 more times.

watchpoints

- The leg action is forward, up, back, down, forward, up . . .
- Lengthen through the leg and out of the hip throughout.
- Keep lifting the waist off the floor and lengthening in the body – long, long waist.
- Your torso should remain absolutely still, do not allow it to roll forward or rock around.
- Don't forget to keep the upper body open; shoulder blades down into your back.
- Do not allow yourself to roll forwards.

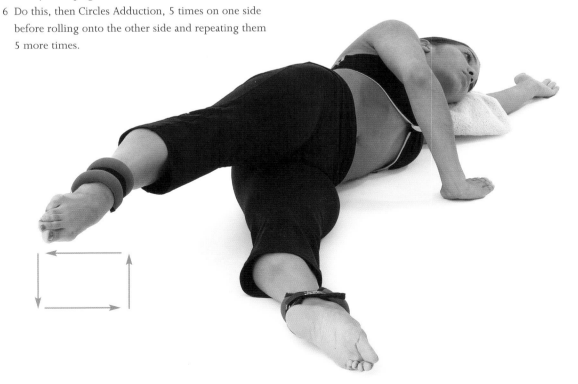

The Exercises

87

Circles Adduction

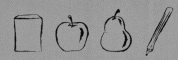

The last exercise worked the thigh and gluteal muscles, but the emphasis was on the outer thigh. This exercise targets the inner thigh and gluteals; it helps prevent wobbly bits. You use the same breathing pattern you learnt in Standing Hundred on page 70.

Equipment

Weights as for Boxes Abduction, plus a large pillow or two. A small flat pillow or a folded towel (optional).

Starting Position

Lie on your left side in a straight line as for Boxes Abduction, but place your top leg on one or two large pillows. The idea is for your pelvis to stay square and not drop forward. The bottom leg is stretched away a little in front of you and turned out from the hip joint. Point or flex the foot, either is fine.

Action

1 Breathe in wide and full to prepare.
2 Keep the leg turned out from the hip, long and straight. Breathe out, zip up and hollow and stay zipped throughout as you slowly raise the underneath leg. Keep lengthening it out of the hip. Do not allow your waist to sink into the floor; keep working it.
3 Breathe in and start to circle the leg forward and up, drawing a small circle the size of a grapefruit.
4 Draw 5 small circles on the in-breath and 5 on the out-breath.
5 Do 5 circles one way then 5 the other way, then lower the leg.
6 Turn over and repeat Boxes Abduction, then Circles Adduction.

watchpoints

- Keep zipping and hollowing throughout.
- Do not let the waist sag; keep lengthening it.
- Check you are moving the leg from the hip, not just from the knee.
- Do not let your foot sickle (curl) round to help you come up further. The action must be in the inside of the thigh.
- Your torso should remain still.
- Check that your upper body stays open, shoulder blades down.
- Do not roll forward.

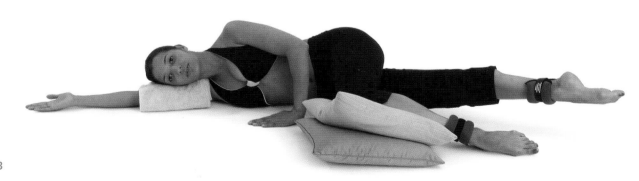

Side Kick Warm Up

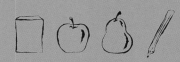

Great for legs and butt! This exercise tones the legs and mobilizes
and strengthens the hips, while maintaining good core stability.
It is a warm-up sequence for your legs and hips. Make sure you keep
yourself firmly anchored, with no movement in your pelvis or hips.

Starting Position

Lie on your right side with your head resting on your right
arm, which is extended in line with your body. You
should be in one straight line, tailbone to elbow. The
pelvis is in neutral. Bend at the hips so your legs are at a
slight angle to your body but still straight. The left leg rests
on the right. Place your left hand on the mat in front of
your chest.

Action

1 Breathe in to prepare.
2 Breathe out, zip up and hollow and stay strongly zipped
  throughout.
3 Breathe in, lift the leg to hip height with the foot softly
  pointed. Kick the leg forward, keeping it at hip level.
  When you reach the end of the sweep forward,
  immediately give a little pulse forward, so that you
  stretch the leg a little further.
4 Breathe out, flex the foot and sweep your leg back,
  keeping it at hip height. Kick as far backwards as you
  can past your anchored leg, and give a little pulse
  backwards at the end of your sweep.
5 Breathe in and point the foot.
6 Do 5 kicks forwards and backwards, breathing in to
  come forwards, breathing out to sweep backwards.
7 Turn over and repeat on the other side.

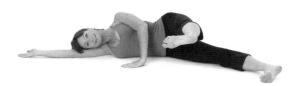

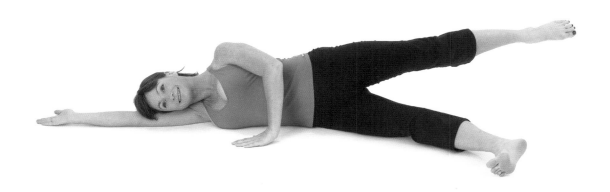

Side Kick Variation

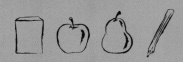

This is a more challenging exercise.

Starting Position

Return to the starting position for Side Kick Warm Up (page 89). Place your right hand behind your head, with the elbow in line with your body. This reduces your base of support and challenges your core stability further.

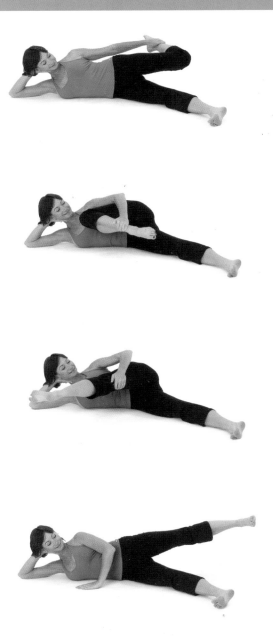

Action

1 Breathe in to prepare.
2 Breathe out, zip up and hollow and stay strongly zipped throughout.
3 Breathe in, stabilize the body and softly point the foot.
4 Breathe out, bend your top knee, bring your heel towards your buttocks and reach back to clasp your ankle. Watch you do not collapse your shoulder, keep it stable.
5 Breathe in and, holding your heel as close to your buttocks as you can, bring your knee up towards your chest, keeping it at hip level. As your knee moves, your foot will come around. Keep pressing your ankle close to your thigh, your thigh close to your chest.
6 When your knee can go no higher, let go of your ankle and clasp the underside of your thigh immediately below your knee.
7 Breathe out, press your thigh towards your chest and slowly straighten your leg. Let your knee move away from your chest a little so you are able to straighten your leg more comfortably.
8 Breathe in when your leg is straight, then sweep it back over the mat at hip level. Put your hand on the floor as soon as your leg passes by to stabilize. When you have kicked as far back as you can, breathe out and clasp your ankle so you can repeat the movement.
9 Do this 3 times, then reverse the movement keeping the same breathing.
10 Turn over and repeat on the other side.

Side Kick Lift

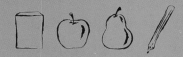

This will test your stability by adding more movements.
It is an advanced exercise.

Starting Position

Remain in the Side Kick position.

Action

1 Breathe in to prepare.

2 Breathe out, zip up and hollow and stay strongly zipped
throughout.

3 Breathe in and kick your top leg with a softly pointed
foot up towards the ceiling.

4 Once you have stretched to your maximum, breathe out
and flex your foot and, with a controlled movement,
bring your leg back to the starting position.

5 Keep the legs straight but not locked. You should not
feel any strain in the neck. Remember to stabilize with
your arms.

6 Repeat 10 times on each side.

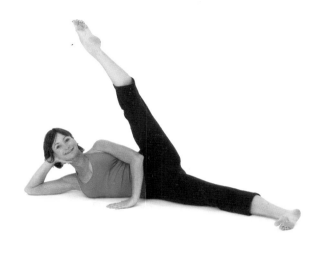

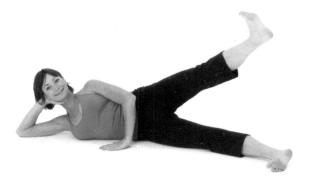

watchpoints for all Side Kicks

1 Keep your trunk anchored firm and motionless.

2 Strong zip throughout.

3 Keep your hips square. Make sure the top hipbone stays
directly over the anchored one.

4 Keep your waistline lifted and long – no collapsing.

5 Keep the elbow you rest on back and in line with your
lower shoulder.

6 Do not let your chest or shoulders sag forward.

7 Keep the movement flowing and controlled.

8 Always keep your leg at hip height as it sweeps backwards or forward across the mat.

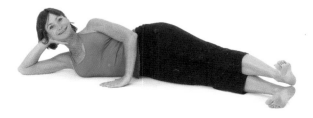

Upright Chair Stretch

This stretch feels wonderful and has the added benefit of strengthening your legs as well as lengthening them and increasing hip and knee joint mobility. It can also be done anywhere.

Equipment

You will need a sturdy chair or stool, one with a wooden seat and good stability!

Starting Position

Stand about 60 cm (2 ft) or more from the chair. Put the ball of one foot flat on the edge of the chair seat. Adjust your position so both legs are straight, your lifted foot is softly pointed, the other foot is in a natural walking position.

Stand upright – imagine there is a wall behind you. Balance evenly and centrally on your standing foot (remember Standing Well on page 67).

Lift your arms up out to the sides to shoulder height. Curve your arms and hands gracefully and bring them forward as though you were holding a light but large beach ball. Feel a lightness and lift in your upper body, but don't lose neutral pelvis. Avoid arching your back or throwing your chest out of line.

Avoid this exercise if you have back problems.

Action

1 Breathe in to prepare and lengthen through the top of the head.
2 Breathe out, zip up and hollow and stay zipped throughout. Keep the back leg straight and your hips square and bend the knee of your raised leg. Your body should stay upright as it moves forward towards the chair. Keep your arms still at shoulder-height holding your ball. When you have gone as far forward as you can, stop. Feel the stretch in your straight leg.
3 Breathe in and hold the stretch.
4 Breathe out and reverse the motion to return to the starting position.
5 Repeat 5 times.

watchpoints

- Your upper body stays light and lifted.
- Keep your back leg straight, hips square.
- Your back hip presses forward.
- Stay zipped throughout.
- Keep your arms gracefully curved, avoid tension creeping into the shoulders by maintaining the distance between the ears and the shoulders.

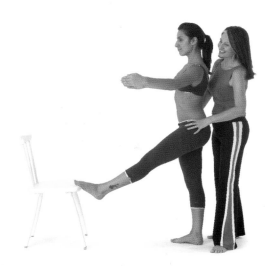
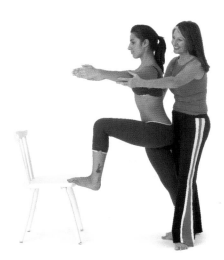

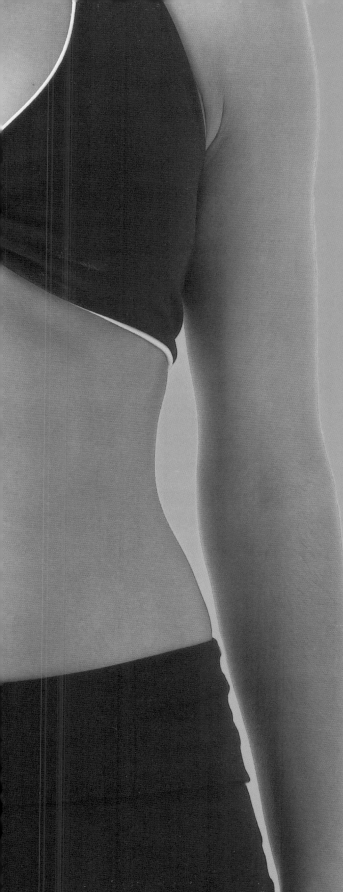

Have you ever wondered why it is that no matter how many stomach exercises you do you still cannot get a flat stomach? We have heard every excuse from having children and operations to food allergies. Of course factors such as these might make achieving a flat stomach difficult but not impossible . . .

Abdominals and Waist

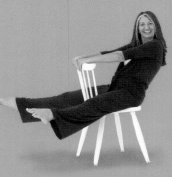

Take me for example. I have had two children, now aged twenty-four and twenty-two. Both were very large babies - nearly ten pounds. I have also had two abdominal operations. Twelve years ago, before I discovered Pilates, I had very poor abdominal control. In fact, I looked as though I was six months pregnant! The secret? Good technique.

Let's look at the anatomy first. You have four abdominal muscles: the superficial rectus abdominis (the six-pack), the internal and external obliques (which define your waist) and underneath these the wrap-around muscle which we have been mentioning throughout the book - the transversus abdominis.

The type of sit-ups commonly done in a gym will work the rectus muscle which creates the famous six-pack. You might consider whether you want a six-pack. It looks great on guys but does it look so good on girls? In fact, the rectus muscle is not nearly as important as you think in achieving good abdominal tone. The muscle fibres of rectus run top to bottom. Think of an old-fashioned corset. In which direction do the fibres of the corset run? They don't run vertically, do they? No, they run horizontally, criss-crossing and wrapping around the trunk like those of transversus.

If you want to achieve the ultimate flat stomach, then you need to focus first on your transversus (with the zip up and hollow and the stability exercises) and then on the obliques (for example with Hip Rolls Variation on page 96). Once you have strengthened these foundation muscles, then you can work on the more superficial muscles, but always, always with the deep transversus muscle engaged as well.

The following section contains powerful abdominal exercises. It is vital that you have practised the basic stability work on pages 41-64 before you attempt these exercises: they simply will not work unless you have. Furthermore, you will need to follow the directions to the letter. Your body will want to cheat: your abdominals may pop up and bulge, your pelvis may slip out of neutral and tilt to the north and either of these negate the benefits of the exercise.

It is better to do five repetitions correctly than a hundred badly.

Remember particularly the instructions for the Basic Curl Up on page 64.

Curl Ups with Frog's Legs

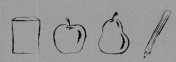

OK, we know it's a silly name, but we believe this is a great way to work your abdominals! You should feel this exercise low down in your abdomen. The leg position will help prevent you tilting your pelvis to north while you curl up.

Starting Position

Lie in the Relaxation Position (page 34). Bring your feet together and allow your knees to open. Check that you have not lost your neutral pelvis; you must not allow your back to arch, it should feel comfortable. Gently release your neck by rolling the head slowly from side to side. Lightly clasp your hands behind your head to cradle and support it (at no point should you pull on your neck). Keep your elbows open just in front of your ears throughout.

Avoid this exercise if you have neck problems.

Action

1 Breathe in wide and full to prepare.
2 Breathe out, zip up and hollow and stay zipped throughout, soften your breastbone, tuck your chin in a little and curl up, breaking from the breastbone. Your stomach must not pop up. Keep the pelvis level and the tailbone down on the floor lengthening away.
3 Breathe in and come up a little higher, but keep your pelvis level and neutral.
4 Breathe out and slowly curl back down, controlling the movement.
5 Repeat 10 times.

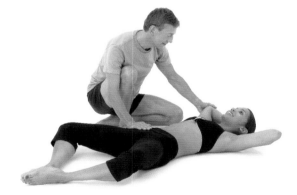

watchpoints

• Stay in neutral, the pelvis tilted neither to north or south (remember the Compass on page 35). The front of the body keeps its length. It's helpful to imagine a strip of sticky tape along the front of the body which should not wrinkle!
• Think of peeling the upper spine bone by bone from the floor.
• Think of the ribs funnelling down towards the waist.
• Keep the chin gently tucked in, this is the cervical nod action you learnt in Neck Rolls and Chin Tucks on page 59. This should help keep your neck released.
• Don't close your elbows as you come up, keep them open but within your peripheral vision.

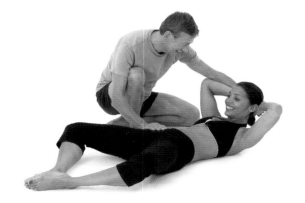

The Exercises

95

Hip Rolls Variation

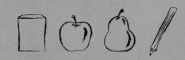

This exercise really works the waist muscles and stretches them too. Having the knee raised adds extra weight which makes you work harder and also helps the stretch. Feels great as well!

Starting Position

Lie in the Relaxation Position (page 34). Bring your feet together, lining up the bones. Have your arms, with palms down, out to the sides just below shoulder height.

Action

1 Breathe in wide and full to prepare.
2 Breathe out, zip up and hollow and stay zipped throughout. Slide your right foot up until it rests beside the left knee.
3 Breathe into your lower ribcage. As you breathe out, roll your head to the right, your knees to the left. Only roll a little way to start with; you can go further each time if it is comfortable. Keep your right shoulder blade down on the floor.
4 Breathe in, then breathe out and use your strong centre to bring the knees back to the starting position, the head moves back as well.
5 Breathe in and slide the foot back to the mat.
6 Repeat 6 times on each side, alternating legs.

Please take advice if you have a disc-related injury.

watchpoints

- Only roll to the same side as the foot still on the floor.
- Keep both sides of the waist long.
- Control the movement from your centre.
- Keep the pelvis still as you slide the foot up into position. It's as if you are doing a Knee Fold (page 48).
- Remember to keep the opposite shoulder blade down on the mat.

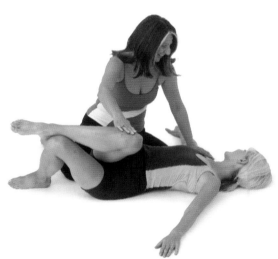

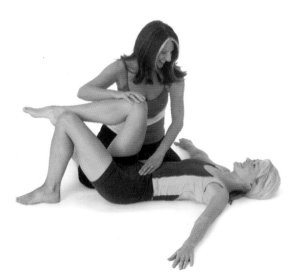

Oblique Roll Ups

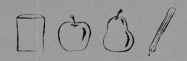

Another great exercise for streamlining the waist. You must be very good at the Basic Curl Up before you try this more challenging intermediate exercise. The idea is to roll across along the line of the shoulder blades, along the lower edge if possible, though this will depend on how far you have curled up in the first place.

Starting Position

Lie in the Relaxation Position (page 34). Lightly clasp your hands behind your head and tuck your chin in gently, as for the Basic Curl Up (page 64).

Action

1 Breathe in wide and full to prepare.
2 Breathe out, zip up and hollow and stay zipped throughout. Curl your upper body up, bringing your left shoulder across towards your right knee. The right elbow stays back. The pelvis stays still, square and stable.
3 Breathe in and roll the upper body across to the centre. Hold the position.
4 Breathe out and roll across the shoulder blades to bring the right shoulder towards the left knee. The pelvis stays square. The abdominals remain hollowed.
5 Breathe in and lower back down.
6 Repeat 6 times, alternating which side you curl up to first.

Avoid this exercise if you have neck problems.

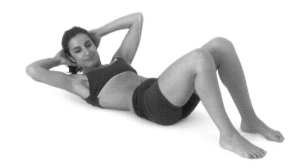

watchpoints

- Keep your chin tucked in gently, your neck released.
- Remember to roll from the lower edge of one shoulder blade to the other.
- Be aware of the movement of your ribcage. It should be rolling too.
- Keep your sides equal in length. There is always a tendency with this exercise to shorten one side of the waist as you come up. Keep the action simple. You are going across at an oblique angle.
- Keep the upper body open, elbows back but in your peripheral view.
- Focus on keeping the pelvis very still; you may find that the opposite hip wants to come up. Stay square and neutral.

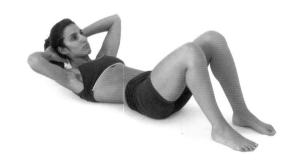

The New Cancan 1 and 2

A fun way to work the abdominals. The action of extending the leg challenges your core muscles.

Once again you have two versions to play with; the second is harder.

Starting Position

Adopt the Relaxation Position (page 34), but have your feet together. Without losing neutral pelvis, come onto your toes. Lightly clasp your hands behind your head. Tuck your chin in gently.

Action

1 Breathe in to the lower ribcage.
2 Breathe out, zip up and hollow and stay zipped throughout. Slowly curl up, simultaneously straightening one leg into the air, keeping the knee in a line with the other knee. The other foot remains on the floor.
3 Breathe in and change legs in a cancan-type action, staying zipped and in neutral. Stomach hollow! One foot always remains in contact with the floor.
4 Repeat 10 times. Stay curled up, your focus down on your stomach.

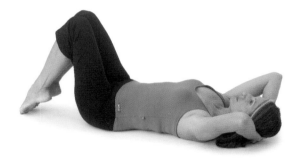

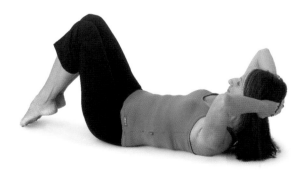

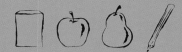

Moving on

As you become stronger you can quicken the pace so you exchange both legs on one breath without returning the foot to the floor.

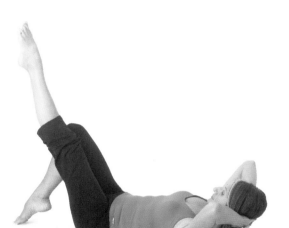

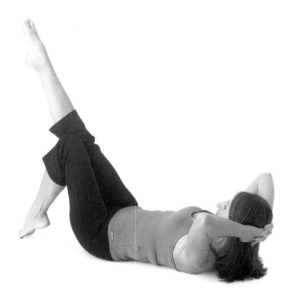

Curled-Up Leg Beats 1 and 2

This is a tough, advanced-level abdominal workout. It requires good core stability, good hamstring length and stamina. It will strengthen your abdominals and your inner-thigh muscles.

Starting Position

Lie in the Relaxation Position (page 34). Zip up and hollow and stay zipped throughout. Double Knee Fold (page 51), connect the inner thighs and feet and lightly hold each leg behind the thigh. Have your elbows open, breastbone soft and shoulder blades down into your back.

Action

1 Breathe in to prepare.
2 Breathe out and, keeping strongly zipped, slowly curl up, simultaneously straightening both legs into the air at an angle of about 90 degrees. Your toes are softly pointed. Your focus is down on your abdominals.
3 Breathe in and turn the legs out from the hips.
4 Breathe out. Still holding the thighs, cross the left leg in front of the right and beat 3 times.

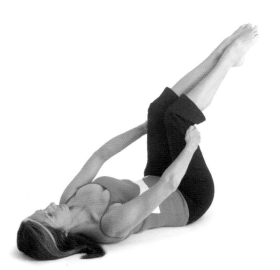

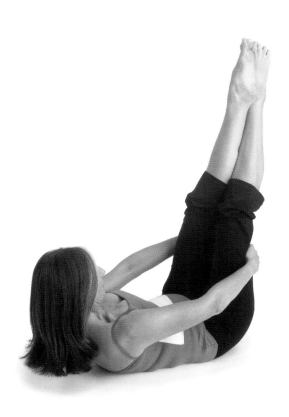

5 Breathe in and separate the legs about 25 cm (10 in) into a splits action.
6 Breathe out and cross them over, right leg in front now and beat 3 times.
7 Breathe in and split again.
8 Repeat up to 6 times.

Version 2

When you are strong enough, you can place the hands behind your head as for a Basic Curl Up (page 64). This is a super-advanced exercise and challenges the abdominals further. Repeat the exercise 5 times, progressing to 12 times.

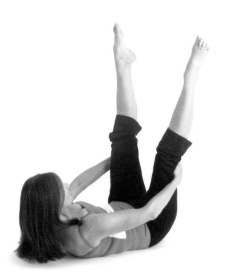

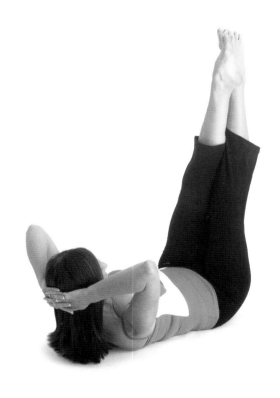

watchpoints

- Your hands are there to guide and steady your legs gently.
- Remember to nod your head before you curl up and, as you stay curled up, keep your focus on your abdomen, which should remain hollow.
- Keep the legs turned out and as straight as possible.
- Stay in neutral, but ensure your back is firmly anchored to the mat by using your core muscles.
- Keep the distance between your ears and your shoulders, shoulder blades down, elbows open.

Diamond Curls (Double Leg Lowers)

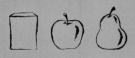

This is another great way to target your lower abdominals.
You will also feel your buttocks working. You can do this exercise
with the hands lightly clasped behind your head (as for the Basic Curl Up),
which is more challenging.

Starting Position

From the Relaxation Position (page 34), Double Knee Fold
(page 51) using a Strong Zip (page 42). Cross your ankles,
right behind left, and open your knees slightly, straightening the legs so they make a long diamond shape. Your legs
will be turned out from the hips but remain above them.
Put your hands on the backs of your thighs, keeping the
elbows up and open in a soft 'C' shape.

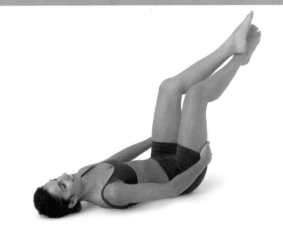

Action

1 Breathe in to prepare.
2 Breathe out, still zipped, nod your head, soften your
   breastbone and slowly curl up, remembering everything
   you learnt for the Basic Curl Up on page 64.
3 Breathe in and hold the position; try to feel your deep
   wrap-around buttock muscles.
4 Breathe out, still zipped, and slowly lower your legs to
   about 45 degrees, still with your hands on your legs.
   The diamond shape will elongate slightly. Feel your
   deep buttock muscles squeezing together. Your focus
   stays on your lower abdominals. Pelvis stays neutral.
5 Breathe in and bring the legs back to the starting
   position, but stay curled up.
6 Repeat 5 times, rest, then repeat 5 times more with the
   ankles crossed the other way.

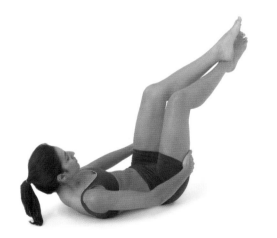

watchpoints

- Stay curled up, keep your focus down on your lower
  abdominals.
- Keep the pelvis neutral, your back anchored to the mat.
  Be particularly careful not to arch your back as your legs
  move away from you.
- Try to feel the action happening in the wrap-around but-
  tock muscles (as in the Pilates Stance on page 68).
- Think of the legs moving away from you rather than
  down.
- Maintain the diamond leg shape.
- Keep your breastbone soft, elbows open and directed
  outwards, neck released.

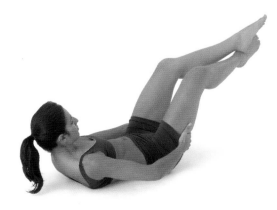

As we have already noted, not many of us look at our back view in the mirror. We tend to worry about our bulging stomachs and flabby thighs, but backs and shoulders are often well down our list of priorities when it comes to the body parts that need work – could this simply be because we can't see them? However, they still need work because strong back muscles are essential to good posture.

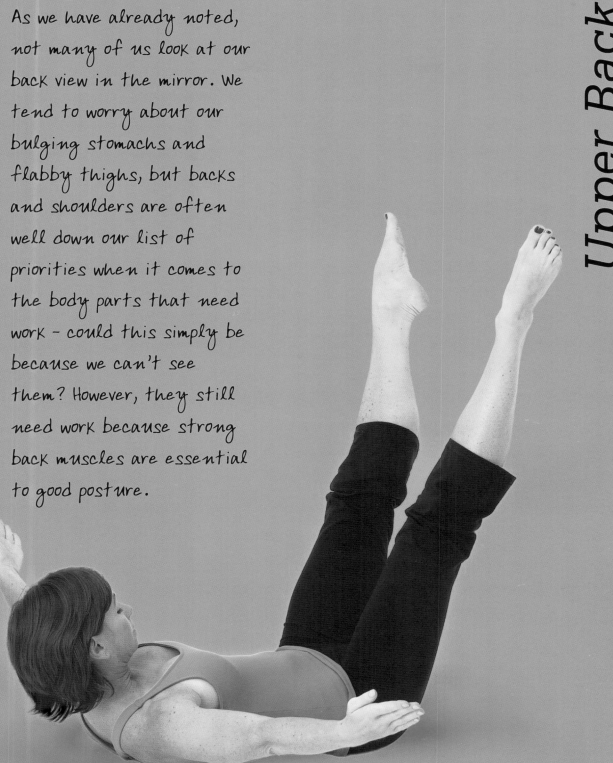

We are often asked if we have any exercises for improving the bust. Because breast tissue is not muscular it is not easy to improve your breasts with exercise. However, you can help change your bust line and you can tackle the problem in two ways: you can strengthen the pectoral muscles which help support the breasts with exercises such as the Standing Hundred (page 70) and the One-Arm Push Ups (page 118); and you can also strengthen the mid-back muscles which help prevent you being round-shouldered, which in turn makes the breasts look saggy. Turn once more to the photo on page 2 of good and bad posture. If you want an instant boob job then stand up tall, open up across your chest and draw your shoulder blades down into your back. The effect is nothing short of miraculous and it is free – well, all you have to do is invest time and effort into strengthening the muscles to hold you there.

Seated Scapular Squeeze

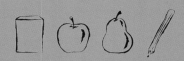

A new position for this Body Control Pilates exercise which is usually done standing. The seated position helps you hinge forward correctly from the hips, which in turn helps you focus on your arm and shoulder action. It is a great way to open the chest and work the upper back and the back of the arms.

Equipment

You will need a sturdy chair which has a narrow back. If it has a wide back you will also be doing an inner-thigh stretch!

Starting Position

Turn the chair around and sit astride it. Sit tall and square. Make sure both feet are firmly planted on the ground. Keep a long back and hinge forward from your hips so your head and back are in a straight line. Look at a spot on the floor in front of you at a distance that keeps the back of your neck free from tension, and the top of the head lengthening away. Take your arms behind you to the sides, with the palms facing upwards.

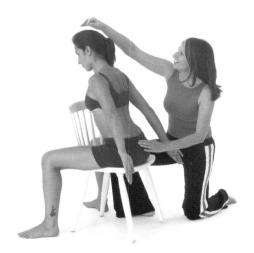

Action

1 Breathe in to prepare and lengthen up through the spine.
2 Breathe out, zip up and hollow, and slide the shoulder blades down before squeezing them together. Your arms are also squeezing towards each other as if the thumbs want to meet.
3 Breathe in and hold.
4 Breathe out and release the arms.
5 Repeat 8 times before returning to upright.

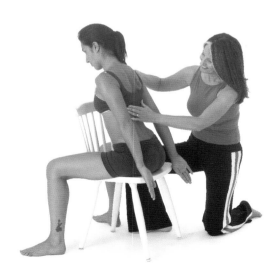

watchpoints

- Keep your gaze on your spot on the floor.
- Check your neck; keep it released and long.
- Think of your tailbone lengthening downwards away from the top of your head.
- Make sure you feel this exercise between the shoulder blades and also in the backs of your upper arms. Do not lock the arms; they are straight but not locked.
- Do not twist the hands and wrists towards each other; they stay as one with the arms.

Simple Diamond Press

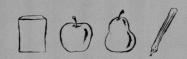

Here you have the Simple Diamond Press and the Diamond Press Salute, which is a more challenging version requiring greater upper-body strength. Focus on the quality of your movement; in this case the movement is simple and minimal but very powerful.

Equipment

A small flat cushion (optional).

Starting Position for Both Versions

Lie on your front in a straight line with your feet hip-width apart and parallel. Create a diamond shape with your arms by placing your fingertips together just above your forehead. Your elbows are open, your shoulder blades relaxed.

> If you are uncomfortable lying on your stomach, place a small flat cushion under your abdomen to support your back.

Action

1 Breathe in and lengthen through the spine.
2 Breathe out, zip up and hollow and stay zipped throughout. Slide the shoulder blades down towards the back of your waist, simultaneously tucking your chin in gently and extending your upper body 3–4 cm (1–2 in) off the floor. Stay looking down at the floor, keeping the back of the neck long. Imagine a cord pulling you from the top of your head. You have to push a little on the elbows, to come up, but this isn't a push-up; make the upper-back muscles work.
3 Breathe in and hold the position. Breathe out and lengthen as you lower back down.
4 Repeat 6 times, then come into the Rest Position (page 58).

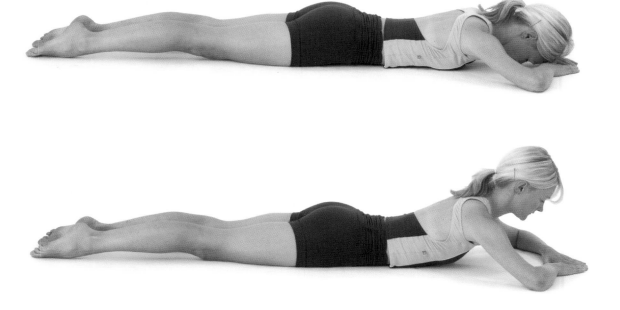

Diamond Press Salute

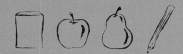

Action

1 Follow points 1 and 2 for the Simple Diamond Press and then breathe in and hold the position, while you bring the back of one hand to touch your forehead (like a salute).
2 Breathe out and lower the hand.
3 Breathe in, still zipped, and salute with the other hand.
4 Breathe out and lower the hand.
5 Breathe in and slowly lengthen as you lower your body back down.
6 Repeat twice, then come back into the Rest Position (page 58).

Moving on

When you are stronger you can bring both hands up at the same time. Even harder is to come up with the hands in the salute position.

watchpoints for both versions

- Keep the lower abdominals drawing back to the spine.
- As you start the movement, imagine you are rolling a marble along the floor with your nose, then follow through, leading with the head, to extend the back gently only as far as the bra line.
- Keep your focus down.
- This is a gentle back extension, so the buttocks can stay relaxed.

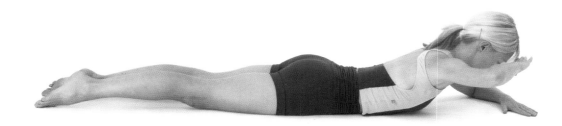

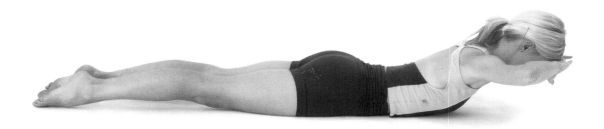

Star Variation

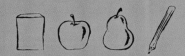

This is similar to the Diamond Press Salute, only this time you lift the leg as well, so you are working both the upper and lower body diagonally. It's great for toning the buttocks and shoulders.

Starting Position

Lie on your front with your legs turned out. The hips just wider than hip-width apart. Fold your right arm so you can rest your forehead on it. Stretch the left arm out so it is just wider than shoulder width. Maintain a distance between the ears and the shoulders. Keep a sense of openness in the upper body.

> If you are uncomfortable lying on your stomach, place a small, flat cushion under your abdomen to support your back.

Action

1 Breathe in to prepare and lengthen through the spine.
2 Breathe out, zip up and hollow and stay zipped throughout. Lengthen first, then simultaneously raise your head, right arm and left leg no more than 5 cm (2 in) off the ground. Stay looking down. The back of the neck is long. Lengthen away from a strong centre. Do not twist in the pelvis, both hip joints stay on the floor.
3 Breathe in and relax.
4 Change hands and repeat with the opposite arm and leg.
5 Repeat 5 times each side.

watchpoints

- Keep both hips on the mat. Remember what you learnt in Star Test (page 83).
- Keep zipping throughout.
- Try to reach out of the hip joint.

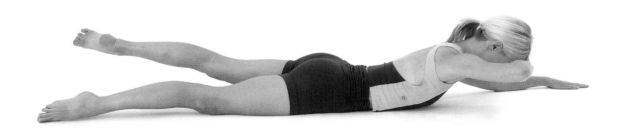

Classical Backstroke Swimming

This exercise tests your core stability and challenges your co-ordination. This is an advanced exercise.

Starting Position

Lie on your back, in neutral, with straight legs, feet together and toes softly pointed. Have your arms down by your sides, just touching the body, with the palms facing down, fingers long.

Action

1 Breathe in to prepare.
2 Breathe out to zip up and hollow and stay strongly zipped throughout.
3 Breathe in and bend your knees to bring your thighs to your chest, at the same time bringing your chin to the chest.
4 Breathe out and bring your knuckles together up under your chin, palms facing away, with your elbows bent and straight out to the side.
5 Breathe in and stretch your arms and legs straight up, keeping them slightly apart and reaching for the ceiling with your fingers and toes. You will lose neutral pelvis.
6 Breathe out, sweep your arms and legs out to the sides and down, keeping your arms in a line with your shoulders.
7 Breathe in, bring your legs together and your hands, palms down, just over your thighs. Stretch your fingers and toes, making them feel long. Your chin is still on your chest. Focus on your centre and hold this position for a moment.
8 Breathe out and return to the position in point 3.
9 Repeat this exercise 5 times.

watchpoints

- Stay strongly zipped throughout.
- Keep your chin on your chest and your focus forward.
- Keep your arms and legs straight but avoid hyperextending them (locking them back).
- Stretch and lengthen out of your hips and shoulders.
- Keep your movements smooth and flowing. Do not rush the exercise; use the breathing to co-ordinate the movements.

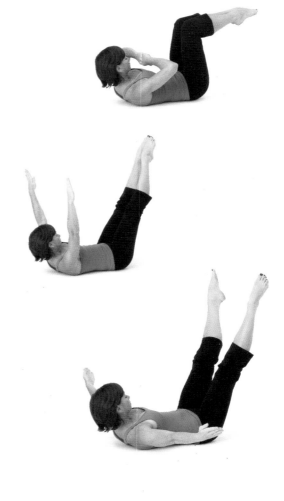

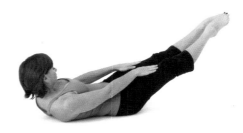

The Exercises

Rowing

A tough, advanced exercise which was part of Joseph Pilates' original mat sequence. You will require excellent core strength and co-ordination to master this exercise – so add it to your routine only when you have the necessary strength and flexibility! Great for your upper back, in fact, great for all of you!

Starting Position

Sit tall with your legs parallel, together and straight out in front of you, with your feet flexed. Have your arms outstretched directly over your thighs, palms facing each other, fingers straight.

> Avoid if you have back or shoulder problems.

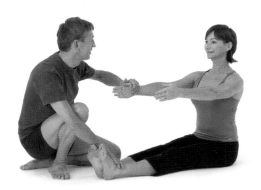

Action

1 Breathe in, sit up out of your hips and lengthen through the crown of your head. Feel yourself anchored to the floor from your heels to the base of your spine.

2 Breathe out, zip up and hollow and stay strongly zipped throughout.

3 Breathe in and start to roll back, tucking your tailbone under, curling your pubic bone towards your chin but still sitting up out of your hips (do not collapse). At the same time bring your chin to your chest, your elbows up and opened out and your knuckles to a point just under your chin. Stop rolling back when your shoulders are about 30 cm (12 in) from the mat.

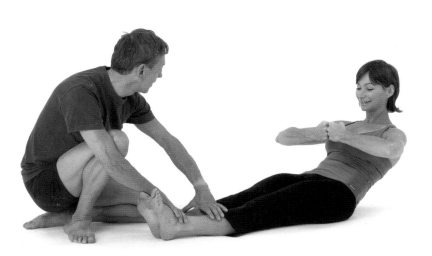

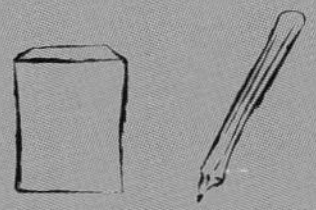

4 Breathe out and extend your hands, which are still
   closed, out to the sides so your arms are out straight in
   a line with each other and your shoulders. Your head
   and body stay still.

5 Once the arms are out straight, extend and stretch your
   fingers and have them facing down to the floor.

6 While breathing in, slowly roll back up, at the same
   time taking your arms around behind you as though
   you were pushing water away with your hands. Rotate
   your wrists so your palms now face the ceiling. Clasp
   your fingers if you can, and keep pressing them
   upwards. This will bring the top of the body forward
   even more.

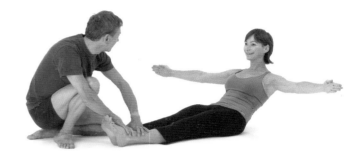

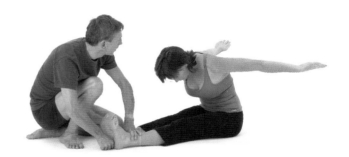

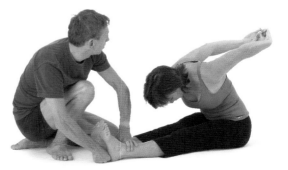

The Exercises

111

Rowing Continued

6 When your clasped hands can go no higher, breathe out, release them and keep rotating your straight arms up and around, into the largest circle your shoulder joint will allow. At the same time, keep curling your head in towards your centre. When your arms have come around, reach out long towards and past your feet.

7 Uncurl into your sitting position and, in the same smooth movement, breathe in and begin to roll down again, bringing your elbows out and closed-up hands under your chin.

8 Repeat this 3 to 5 times.

Reminder on the Breathing

- Breathe in to roll back.
- Breathe out to stretch the arms out to the sides.
- Breathe in to roll back up, push the water away and clasp the fingers.
- Breathe out to circle the arms, curl the head in and then uncurl.
- Breathe in to roll back again.

watchpoints

- Stay strongly zipped throughout.
- Keep your legs straight and your feet flexed; your heels remain on the floor throughout.
- Keep your chin tucked in to your chest throughout.
- Try not to grip around your hips. Use your buttock muscles instead.
- Really stretch and reach right out of your shoulders with your arms.
- When you rotate your arms, do so in the same way as you learnt with the Cleopatra on page 72.
- Make the biggest circle you can without losing stability.

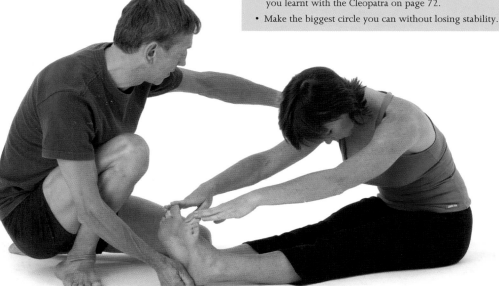

Do you dread summer and those wonderful little strappy dresses you dare not wear because your upper arms are flabby? Read on . . .

Shoulders and Arms

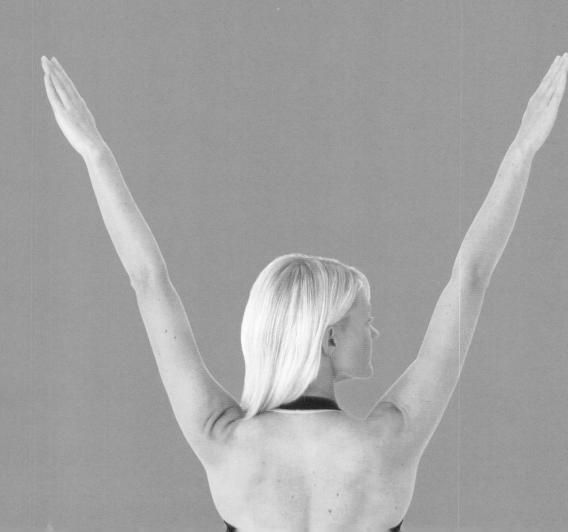

Side Twist

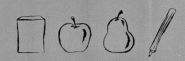

This works the upper body, the sides, the arms and the waist. It was hard to decide which section it should go in. It is great for all-over strength! Think long and strong.

Starting Position

Sit on your left hip with your legs bent. Have them a comfortable distance from your body. Prop up your upper body with your left arm. Your left hand is on the floor to the side and in front of you with the fingertips pointing to eleven o'clock (see photo). Your right hand is resting softly in front of you. Move your right leg so the sole of your right foot is on the mat, close to and in front of the ankle of the left leg. Your right foot points to about two o'clock.

Action

1 Breathe in wide and full to prepare and lengthen through the spine.
2 Breathe out, zip up and hollow and stay zipped throughout. Lift your right hip up towards the ceiling by pushing into your right foot. The left knee stays down. At the same time, float the right arm up and over your head to reach across to the top corner of the room.
3 Breathe in and hold the stretch.
4 Breathe out and slowly lower the body to the mat, circling the right arm back down.
5 Repeat up to 5 times on each side.

Avoid this one if you have shoulder, arm or neck problems.

watchpoints

- Really push into the whole of the front foot.
- Try to connect with the muscles under the shoulder blades and armpits.
- The supporting arm should be straight but not locked.
- Maintain a distance between your ears and your shoulders.
- When you have lifted your body from the mat, do not let the pelvis roll forward.
- It helps to imagine a large thick strap wrapped around your hips lifting you up towards the ceiling.
- Your eye focus is forward throughout.

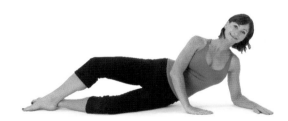

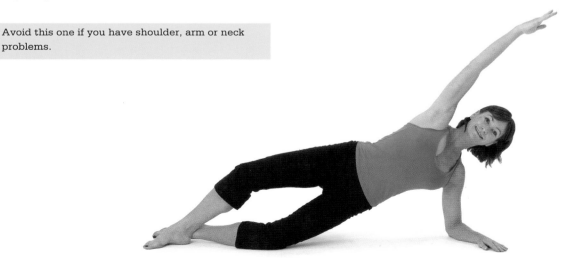

Threading a Needle with Arm Openings

The combination of the two exercises, Threading a Needle and Arm Openings makes for a more demanding but very satisfying movement. It will strengthen your arms and also work the waist muscles and well as opening the chest.

Starting Position
Come onto all fours, hands under shoulders, knees under hips, long neck and the head in good alignment with the spine, which should have its natural curves. Your focus is down on the floor.

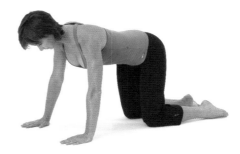

Action
1 Breathe in wide and full and transfer your weight onto the left hand. Avoid moving your feet.
2 Breathe out, zip up and hollow and stay zipped throughout. Slide the back of the right hand along the mat under the left arm, which bends. Your head follows the movement. If comfortable, it can come to rest on the floor.
3 Breathe in and slide your hand back but do not stop as you . . .
4 Breathe out and open the chest and arm to the ceiling, keeping your focus on your hand. You are still zipping. Stretch through your fingers, but do not over-reach – it should feel good.
5 Breathe in and hold the position.
6 Breathe out to return to the starting position and repeat the entire movement.
7 Repeat 4 times on each side, alternating.

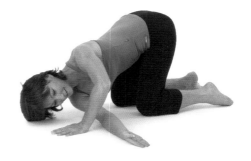

Moving on
Start by lifting the arm to the ceiling first.

watchpoints

- Think of the ribcage moving on the spine to get a maximum stretch.
- Your core muscles must continue to support your spine throughout.
- The movement should be controlled but flowing.
- Keep the weight on the whole of the supporting hand, not just the heel of the hand, but do not press down either into the hand or the knees.
- Be aware of your focus, it will help with your neck alignment.

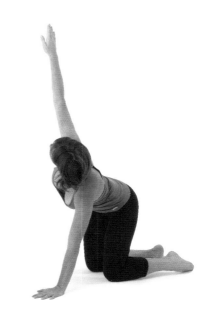

The Exercises

115

Axe

A good upper-body workout. Ideally, this exercise is done on a bench because you can get a greater range of motion. It works both arm and shoulder muscles and prepares you for any Pilates exercise which requires upper-body strength.

Equipment

One hand-held weight of up to 5 kg (10 lb). As both hands are holding the weight, if your technique is good, you can use a heavier weight. A plump cushion (optional).

Starting Position

Lie in the Relaxation Position (page 34), put the cushion between your knees. This helps keep your pelvis stable. Hold the weight in both hands. The elbows are bent above your ribcage at an angle of about 90 degrees. Put the cushion between your knees and gently squeeze it throughout the exercise.

Action

1 Breathe in to prepare, then breathe out, zip up and hollow and stay zipped throughout.

2 Breathe in and lower the weight back behind the head towards the floor. Keep the same shape with the elbows and wrists. The movement originates from the shoulders. Keep your ribcage down.

3 Breathe out and hinge the weight back to the starting position.

4 Repeat up to 10 times.

watchpoints

- Keep the action smooth and controlled both ways: down and up.
- Make the movement from the shoulder joints.
- Keep your shoulder blades down into your back.
- Keep your upper shoulders and neck released.
- Keep squeezing the cushion to work the inner thighs, but stay in neutral pelvis.

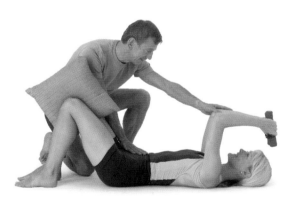

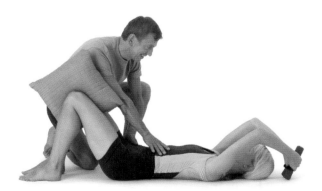

Boxing

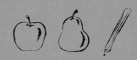

Try this exercise without the weights first of all. It is a very good workout for the arms and shoulders with the added bonus that you are also working the thighs.

Equipment
Two hand-held weights of 0.5 kg (1 lb) each.

Starting Position
Stand tall, feet hip-width apart in parallel. Hinge forward from the hips, keeping your back straight (but still with its natural curves). Look down and find a spot to focus on that keeps the length in the back of your neck. You should look as though you are skiing downhill. Have your elbows bent close to your body, your hands making fists with the weights as if about to box someone!

watchpoints

- Keep your movements slow and controlled.
- Fully extend the punching arm but do not lock it back.

Action
1 Breathe in and lengthen from the crown of your head to your tailbone.
2 Breathe out, zip up and hollow and stay zipped throughout. Slowly punch the air with your right hand, simultaneously taking the left hand back and turning the wrist so that the palm faces upwards. The punch arm is in a line with your ear, the back arm continues the same line.
3 Breathe in and reverse the arms, keeping them close to your body. Breathe out as the punching arm fully extends.
4 Repeat 10 times.

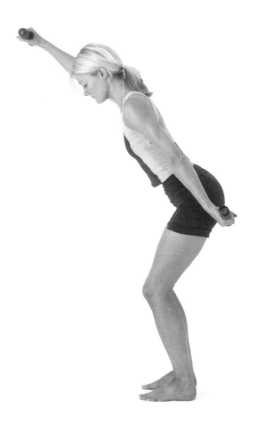

One-Arm Push Ups

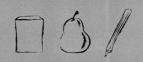

This exercise really builds upper-body strength. It works the pectorals, triceps and the muscles below the shoulder blades. It is a great way to sculpt your upper arms without the use of equipment because you are using your body's own weight against gravity.

This is a good preparation exercise for Stretching Mermaid.

Starting Position

Lie on your left side with your legs slightly bent. Place your right hand on the floor in front of you at about chest height, palm down (you may have to move the hand up or down in order to get the leverage to push up). Your left arm rests across your chest (this is basically to get it out of the way!).

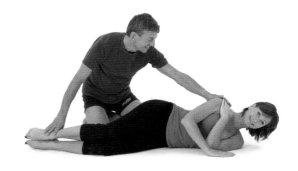

Action

1 Breathe in to prepare, lengthen through the body and try to connect with the muscles below the shoulder blades which wrap round the ribcage under the armpit.

2 Breathe out, zip up and hollow and stay zipped throughout. Press down through the right hand, straightening the right arm so the upper body lifts. You will naturally twist slightly as you do this.

3 Breathe in and hold.

4 Breathe out, still zipping and slowly, slowly, slowly lower.

5 Repeat up to 8 times on each side.

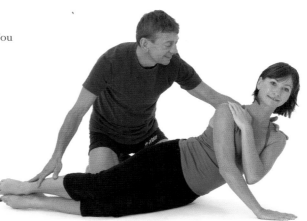

watchpoints

- Did we mention that you lower slowly? The slower you lower the harder you have to work!
- Remember that you may have to adjust the position of your push-up hand to get leverage.
- If you are still finding it difficult, try adjusting your leg position.
- Control the movement; work with the breath.
- Do not allow your neck or the muscles on the top of your shoulders to overwork.
- Try to keep good alignment of the neck on the spine.

Stretching Mermaid Stages 1, 2 and 3

This is a big stretch which works the arms and the side and back muscles.
We've excelled ourselves this time in the number of action points.
Read through the directions several times or think about recording them on tape.

We have broken the exercise down into three stages as it is a lot to learn in one go. Practise Stage 1 several times before attempting Stage 2, and do the same awith Stage 2 before trying Stage 3.

Most people find they are more flexible on one side, so just work within your comfort range. When you roll, you roll your upper body forward – try to remember the action from Oblique Roll Ups (page 97).

Starting Position

Kneel down and lengthen up through the spine. Slowly go over to one side so you are sitting on your right hip. Have both your legs bent so your feet are next to your bottom and your left hand is resting on the left shin. Both hips and shoulders should be on the same plane. Adjust your posture if necessary for a more comfortable sitting position. Keep lengthening up through the crown of the head. The fingers of your right hand should just be touching the mat so you feel totally balanced.

Action for Stage 1

1 Breathe in to prepare.
2 Breathe out, zip up and hollow and stay zipped throughout.
3 Breathe in and turn your head to the right, simultaneously lifting up your right arm in a long sweeping movement from the side. Place your hand on the back of the skull with your elbow bent. Wrap your whole arm around the head.
4 Breathe out and stretch, bending towards your left side.

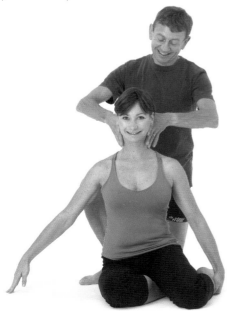

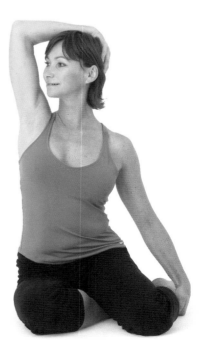

Stretching Mermaid Stage 2

5 Breathe in and hold the position.

6 Breathe out and gently go deeper into the stretch by lengthening through the elbow to the left. Do not compress your side.

7 Breathe in and hold the position again.

8 Breathe out and allow the right elbow and shoulder to slightly roll in, still stretching to the left. Keep your buttocks anchored.

9 Breathe in and with one flowing movement return the elbow and shoulder to face front.

10 While breathing out, unfold the right arm as you turn the head to face front and place the right hand on the floor on the right side.

11 Repeat 2–3 times then change sides.

Action for Stage 2

Follow action points 1–10 above, then move smoothly into action point 12.

12 Still breathing out and placing your right hand on the floor on the right side, slide the hand a little further out to the right side and bend the elbow so the forearm is on the floor, with the palm facing down.

13 Breathe in and simultaneously lift your left arm bringing it close to your left ear, stretching and reaching through your fingertips.

14 Breathe out and stretch, reaching with your left hand towards the right side and keeping the right side of the ribcage away from the floor.

15 Breathe in and hold the position.

16 Breathe out and stretch a little further, reaching with your left hand to the right.

17 Breathe in wide and full into your ribs, holding your position once again.

18 Breathe out and bring the left arm back in line with the body and at the same time push with the right arm to lift upright back to the starting position.

19 Repeat 2–3 times, then change to the other side.

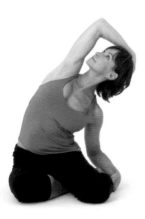

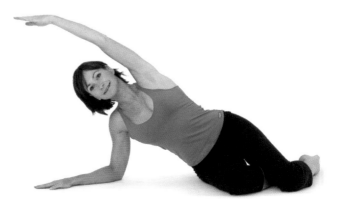

Stretching Mermaid Stages 3

Action for Stage 3

Amalgamate stages 1 and 2 (action points 1–10, 12–17) to make one flowing exercise, and then:

20 Breathe out and allow the left arm to drop slightly forwards, stretch a little more keeping the ribcage closed.

21 Breathe in and bring the left arm back in line with the body. Breathe out and at the same time push with the right arm to lift upright back to the starting position.

22 Repeat 2–3 times, then change to the other side.

watchpoints

- Do not stretch to a point where it is painful or unpleasant.
- Keep your ribcage intact and integrated with your waist at all times. Do not let the ribs stick out.
- Keep your shoulders away from the ears.
- Stay strongly zipped.
- Watch your neck and head alignment – it should look and feel natural.
- Start with the small stretches, then progress to the deep stretches.
- Do not lock your elbows or fingers and keep the movements flowing.
- Do not sink into your joints – keep lengthening out of your hips.

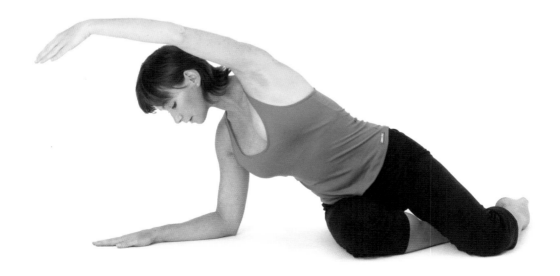

The Exercises

On the following pages we have laid out a four-week programme for each body shape.

If you are still uncertain of your body shape or if you simply wish to do a general workout we suggest you follow the pear-shaped programme. If you wish to spread your programme over more than four weeks, then you may reduce your number of workouts to three a week, but no less or you will not see the benefits.

We have designed five workouts per body shape. Each workout is approximately 45 minutes long and is perfectly balanced. The workouts get progressively harder and are devised to build your strength and flexibility gradually and to teach you new skills. You must be familiar with (and competent with) all the basics on pages 34-64 before you start the main programme. This is non-negotiable! Your four-week programme starts after you have mastered these basics skills.

When you are ready to begin the main programme, you should use the first three workouts designed for your body shape in rotation for the first two weeks. At the start of week three you can add workouts 4 and 5. They will be more challenging. If you do not feel comfortable with the harder exercises, then continue with your first three workouts. If you are happy to include workouts 4 and 5, then follow the schedule given. You can, of course, start adding just a few of the more challenging exercises to workouts 1, 2 and 3.

Some of the exercises in this book have different levels of difficulty. If no level is mentioned in the workouts, start with the Stage 1 version and progress to the other levels when you feel ready. This may, of course take more than four weeks. If a level is indicated but feels too difficult, then stick to the easier level until you are stronger. It will be counter-productive to strain your body.

Where the exercises require the use of hand-held weights, start with the lightest weights and work up. Good technique is always the baseline. For leg weights, try the exercises without weights first, then add 0.5 kg (1 lb) weights working up to 1 kg (2.5 lb) per weight.

Pear Shape 🍐   Workout 1

You must learn the basic exercises
on pages 34–64 before you begin.

Weeks 1 and 2

For your first two weeks please use
workouts 1, 2 and 3 in rotation.

Do not forget to include your
recommended aerobic activities (page 24).

- Thirty accumulative minutes a day
  (brisk walking) at least five times
  a week.
- At least 2 x 30 minutes of continuous
  aerobic activity per week.

Spine Curls	p. 81	
Leg Sweeps	p. 78	
Basic Curl Up	p. 64	
Hip Rolls Variation	p. 96	
Oyster 1	p. 84	
Standing on One Leg	p. 69	
Leg Shaper	p. 76	
Cleopatra	p. 72	
Side Twist	p. 114	
Axe	p. 116	
Dart Stage 2	p. 57	
Star Test	p. 83	
Rest Position	p. 58	

Workout 2

Pilates Stance	p. 68	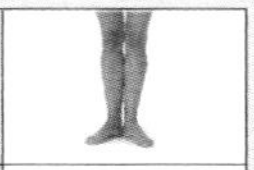
Standing Arm Openings	p. 74	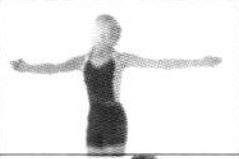
Standing Hundred	p. 70	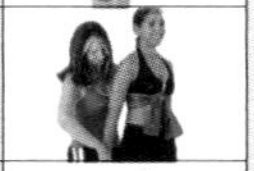
Knee Folds with Openings	p. 49	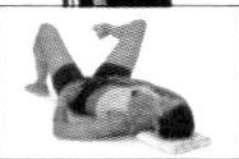
Curl Ups with Frog's Legs	p. 95	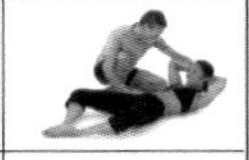
Shoulder Reach 2	p. 55	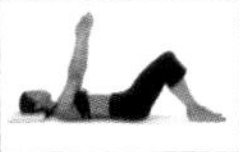
Seated Scapular Squeeze	p. 105	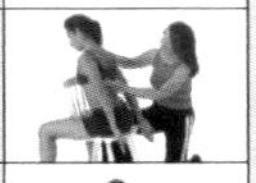
Axe	p. 116	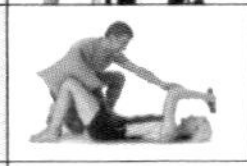
Oyster 2	p. 84	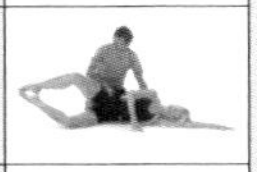
Simple Diamond Press	p. 106	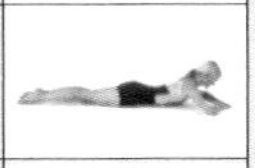
Threading a Needle with Arm Openings	p. 115	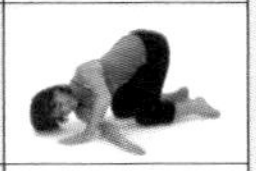
Rest Position	p. 58	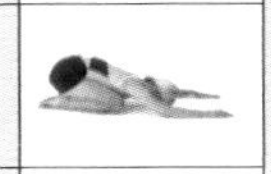
Spine Curls	p. 81	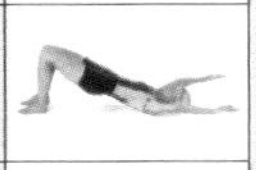
Arm Circles	p. 80	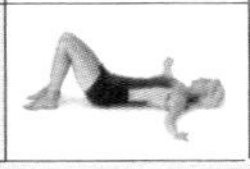

Workout 3

Leg Sweeps	p. 78	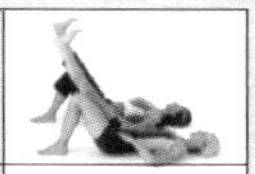
Curl Ups with Frog's Legs	p. 95	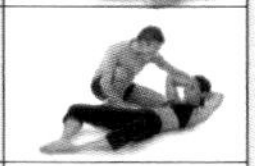
Diamond Curls	p. 102	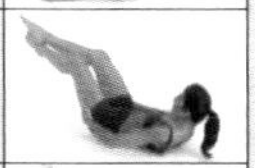
New Cancan 1	p. 98	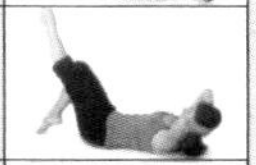
Hip Rolls Variation	p. 96	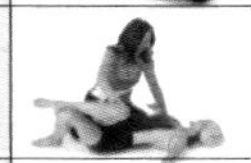
Boxes Abduction (no weights)	p. 86	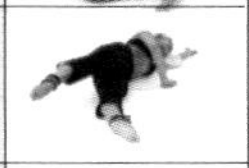
Circles Adduction (no weights)	p. 88	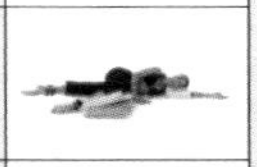
Side Twist	p. 114	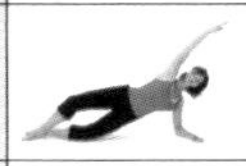
Dart Stage 2	p. 57	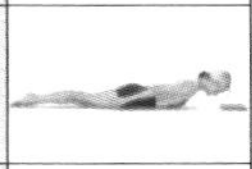
Rest Position	p. 58	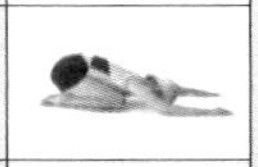
Cleopatra	p. 72	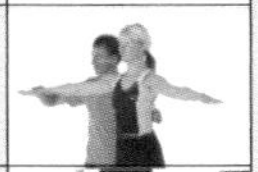
Leg Shaper	p. 76	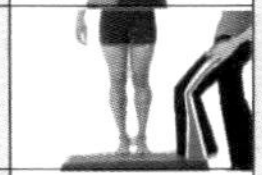
Boxing	p. 117	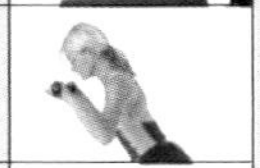
Full Starfish	p. 63	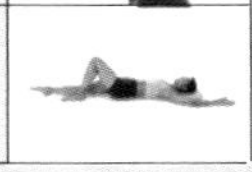

The Workouts

125

Workout 4

Weeks 3 and 4

The following two workouts may now be added into your schedule if you feel strong enough.

Workout 5

When you feel ready, add the exercises below – this may not be for several months. Curled-Up Leg Beats page 101, Side Kick Lift page 91 and Rowing page 110.

Exercise	Page	
Spine Curls with Arm Circles	p. 80	
Double Knee Folds	p. 51	
Basic Curl Up	p. 64	
Diamond Curls	p. 102	
Oblique Roll Ups	p. 97	
One-Arm Push Ups	p. 118	
Oyster 1 and 2	p. 84	
Upright Chair Stretch	p. 92	
Seated Scapular Squeeze	p. 105	
Bottom Worker	p. 82	
Cleopatra	p. 72	
Boxing	p. 117	
Diamond Press Salute	p. 107	
Threading a Needle with Arm Openings	p. 115	
Rest Position	p. 58	

Exercise	Page	
Standing Arm Openings	p. 74	
Leg Shaper	p. 76	
Curl Ups with Frog's Legs	p. 95	
New Cancan 1 (or 2 if possible)	p. 98	
Oblique Roll Ups	p. 97	
Hip Rolls Variation	p. 96	
Stretching Mermaid Stage 1	p. 119	
Axe	p. 116	
Boxes Abduction (with weights)	p. 86	
Circles Adduction (with weights)	p. 88	
Dart Stage 2	p. 57	
Star Variation	p. 108	
Rest Position	p. 58	

Apple Shape Workout 1

You must learn the basic exercises
on pages 34–64 before you begin.

Weeks 1 and 2

For your first two weeks please use
workouts 1, 2 and 3 in rotation.
Do not forget to include your
recommended aerobic sessions.

- Thirty accumulative minutes per day
  (brisk walking).
- At least 2 x 30 minutes of continuous
  aerobic activity per week.

Full Starfish	p. 63	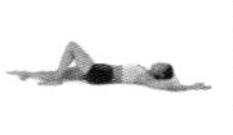
Basic Curl Up	p. 64	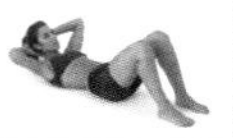
Spine Curls	p. 81	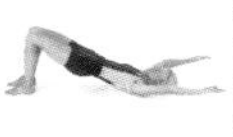
Arm Circles	p. 80	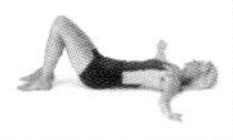
Hip Rolls Variation	p. 96	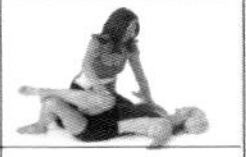
Star Test	p. 83	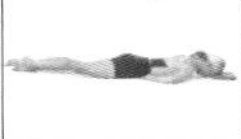
Simple Diamond Press	p. 106	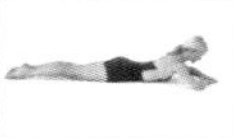
Dart Stage 2	p. 57	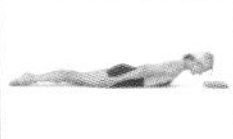
Rest Position	p. 58	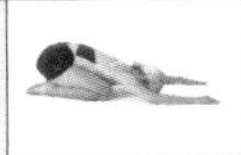
Axe	p. 116	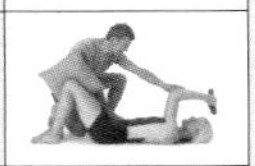
Side Twist	p. 114	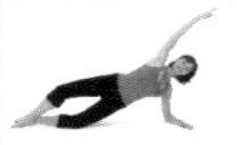
Cleopatra	p. 72	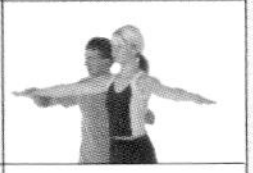
Standing Arm Openings	p. 74	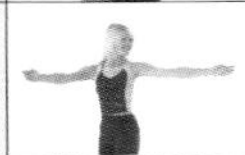
Leg Shaper	p. 76	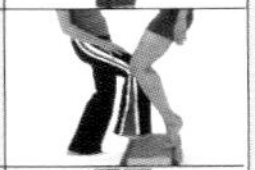
Standing on One Leg	p. 69	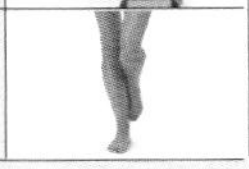

Workout 2

Knee Folds with Openings	p. 49	
Leg Sweeps	p. 78	
Shoulder Reach 2	p. 55	
Curl Ups with Frog's Legs	p. 95	
Hip Rolls Variation	p. 96	
Oyster 1 and 2	p. 84	
Seated Scapular Squeeze	p. 105	
Upright Chair Stretch	p. 92	
Standing Hundred	p. 70	
Boxing	p. 117	
Leg Shaper	p. 76	
Dart Stage 2	p. 57	
Threading a Needle with Arm Openings	p. 115	
Rest Position	p. 58	

Workout 3

Pilates Stance	p. 68	
Cleopatra	p. 72	
Spine Curls	p. 81	
New Cancan 1	p. 98	
Hip Rolls Variation	p. 96	
Double Knee Fold	p. 51	
Diamond Curls	p. 102	
Full Starfish	p. 63	
Side Twist	p. 114	
Boxes Abduction (no weights)	p. 86	
Circles Adduction (no weights)	p. 88	
Arm Circles	p. 80	
Axe	p. 116	
Diamond Press Saulte	p. 107	
Rest Position	p. 58	

Workout 4

Week 3 and 4
The following two workouts may be added into your schedule if you feel strong enough.

Workout 5

When you feel ready, add the exercises below – this may not be for several months. Curled-Up Leg Beats page 101, Side Kick Lift page 91 and Rowing page 110.

Exercise	Page	
Spine Curls with Arm Circles	p. 80	
Oblique Roll Ups	p. 97	
One-Arm Push Ups	p. 118	
Oyster 2	p. 84	
Boxes Abduction (with weights)	p. 86	
Circles Adduction (with weights)	p. 88	
Diamond Press Salute	p. 107	
Threading a Needle with Arm Openings	p. 115	
Rest Position	p. 58	
Stretching Mermaid Stage 1 (2 and 3 when able)	p. 119	
Standing Hundred	p. 70	
Upright Chair Stretch	p. 92	
Standing on One Leg	p. 69	

Exercise	Page	
Leg Sweeps	p. 78	
Curl Ups with Frog's Legs	p. 95	
New Cancan 1 (2 when able)	p. 98	
Diamond Curls	p. 102	
Hip Rolls Variation	p. 96	
Bottom Worker	p. 82	
Stretching Mermaid Stage 1 (2 and 3 when able)	p. 119	
Leg Shaper	p. 76	
Cleopatra	p. 72	
Boxing	p. 117	
Axe	p. 116	
Star Variation	p. 108	
Rest Position	p. 58	

Rectangular Shape   Workout 1

You must learn the basic exercises on pages 34–64 before you begin.

Weeks 1 and 2

For your first two weeks please use workouts 1, 2 and 3 in rotation.

Do not forget to include your recommended 30 accumulative minutes per day of aerobic activity at least five times a week. You may also add 2 x 30 minutes of continuous aerobic activity each week if you wish.

Exercise	Page	
Spine Curls	p. 81	
Arm Circles	p. 80	
Knee Folds with Openings	p. 49	
Basic Curl Up	p. 64	
Hip Rolls Variation	p. 96	
Oyster 1	p. 84	
Side Twist	p. 114	
Cleopatra	p. 72	
Standing Hundred	p. 70	
Standing on One Leg	p. 69	
Seated Scapular Squeeze	p. 105	
Dart Stage 2	p. 57	
Star Test	p. 83	
Rest Position	p. 58	
Relaxation Position	p. 34	

Workout 2

Leg Sweeps	p. 78	
Curl Ups with Frog's Legs	p. 95	
Double Knee Folds	p. 51	
Diamond Curls	p. 102	
Oyster 2	p. 84	
Stretching Mermaid Stage 1	p. 119	
Standing Arm Openings	p. 74	
Upright Chair Stretch	p. 92	
Boxes Abduction (weights optional)	p. 86	
Circles Adduction (weights optional)	p. 88	
Dart Stage 2	p. 57	
Threading a Needle with Arm Openings	p. 115	
Rest Position	p. 58	

Workout 3

Standing on One Leg	p. 69	
Cleopatra	p. 72	
Leg Sweeps	p. 78	
Spine Curls with Arm Circles	p. 80	
Curl Ups with Frog's Legs	p. 95	
Oblique Roll Ups	p. 97	
Oyster 2	p. 84	
Charleston	p. 85	
Bottom Worker	p. 82	
Star Variation	p. 108	
Threading a Needle with Arm Openings	p. 115	
Rest Position	p. 58	
Side Twist	p. 114	
Seated Scapular Squeeze	p. 105	
Upright Chair Stretch	p. 92	
Relaxation Position	p. 34	

Workout 4

Weeks 3 and 4
The following two workouts may now be added into your schedule if you feel strong enough.

Shoulder Reach 2	p. 55	
Knee Folds with Openings	p. 49	
New Cancan 2	p. 98	
Diamond Curls	p. 102	
Hip Rolls Variation	p. 96	
Boxes Abduction	p. 86	
Circles Adduction	p. 88	
Charleston	p. 85	
Diamond Press Salute	p. 107	
Rest Position	p. 58	
Stretching Mermaid Stage 1 (2 and 3 when able)	p. 119	
Standing Hundred	p. 70	
Standing on One Foot	p. 69	

Workout 5

When you feel ready, add the exercises below – this may not be for several months. Curled-Up Leg Beats page 101, Side Kick Lift page 91 and Rowing page 110.

Double Knee Fold	p. 51	
Spine Curls with Arm Circles	p. 80	
Curl Ups with Frog's Legs	p. 95	
Full Starfish	p. 63	
Oblique Roll Ups	p. 97	
Threading a Needle with Arm Openings	p. 115	
Cleopatra	p. 72	
Leg Shaper	p. 76	
Dart Stage 2	p. 57	
Star Variation	p. 108	
Side Twist	p. 114	
Rest Position	p. 58	
Relaxation Position	p. 34	

Pencil Shape Workout 1

You must learn the basic exercises
on pages 34–64 before you begin.

Weeks 1 and 2

For your first two weeks please use
workouts 1, 2 and 3 in rotation.

Do not forget to include your
recommended 30 accumulative minutes per
day of aerobic activity at least five times
a week. Add at least one session of longer
aerobic activity per week.

Full Starfish	p. 63	
Spine Curls	p. 81	
Arm Circles	p. 80	
Basic Curl Ups	p. 64	
Hip Rolls Variation	p. 96	
Knee Folds with Openings	p. 49	
Side Twist	p. 114	
Axe	p. 116	
Oyster 1	p. 84	
Pilates Stance	p. 68	
Leg Shaper	p. 76	
Standing Arm Openings	p. 74	
Star Test	p. 83	
Dart Stage 2	p. 57	
Rest Position	p. 58	

Workout 2

Pilates Stance	p. 68	
Standing Hundred	p. 70	
Cleopatra	p. 72	
Leg Sweeps	p. 78	
Knee Folds with Openings	p. 49	
Shoulder Reach 2	p. 55	
Oyster 1 and 2	p. 84	
Seated Scapular Squeeze	p. 105	
Simple Diamond Press	p. 106	
Threading a Needle with Arm Openings	p. 115	
Rest Position	p. 58	
Boxing	p. 117	
Relaxation Position	p. 34	

Workout 3

Double Knee Folds	p. 51	
Spine Curls with Arm Circles	p. 80	
Basic Curl Ups	p. 64	
Full Starfish	p. 63	
Diamond Curls	p. 102	
Hip Rolls Variation	p. 96	
Boxes Abduction (no weights)	p. 86	
Circles Adduction (no weights)	p. 88	
Side Twist	p. 114	
Dart Stage 2	p. 57	
Rest Position	p. 58	
Leg Shaper	p. 76	
Cleopatra	p. 72	
Standing on One Leg	p. 69	

Workout 4

Weeks 3 and 4
The following two workouts can now be added into your schedule if you feel strong enough.

Workout 5

When you feel ready, add the exercises below – this may not be for several months. Curled-Up Leg Beats page 101, Side Kick Lift page 91 and Rowing page 110

Exercise	Page	
Standing Hundred	p. 70	
Threading a Needle with Arm Openings	p. 115	
Rest Position	p. 58	
Curl Ups with Frog's Legs	p. 95	
New Cancan 1 (2 when able)	p. 98	
Bottom Worker	p. 82	
One-Arm Push Ups	p. 118	
Boxes Abduction (with weights)	p. 86	
Circles Adduction (with weights)	p. 88	
Oyster 2 and Charleston	pp. 84 and 85	
Stretching Mermaid Stage 1 (2 and 3 when able)	p. 119	
Star Variation	p. 108	
Rest Position	p. 58	

Exercise	Page	
Shoulder Reach 2	p. 55	
Spine Curls with Arm Circles	p. 80	
Leg Sweeps	p. 78	
Curls Ups with Frog's Legs	p. 95	
Oblique Roll Ups	p. 97	
Diamond Curls	p. 102	
Hip Rolls Variation	p. 96	
Side Twist	p. 114	
Bottom Worker	p. 82	
Dart Stage 2	p. 57	
Rest Position	p. 58	
Oyster 1 and 2	p. 84	
Boxing	p. 117	
Axe	p. 116	
Relaxation Position	p. 34	

The Workouts

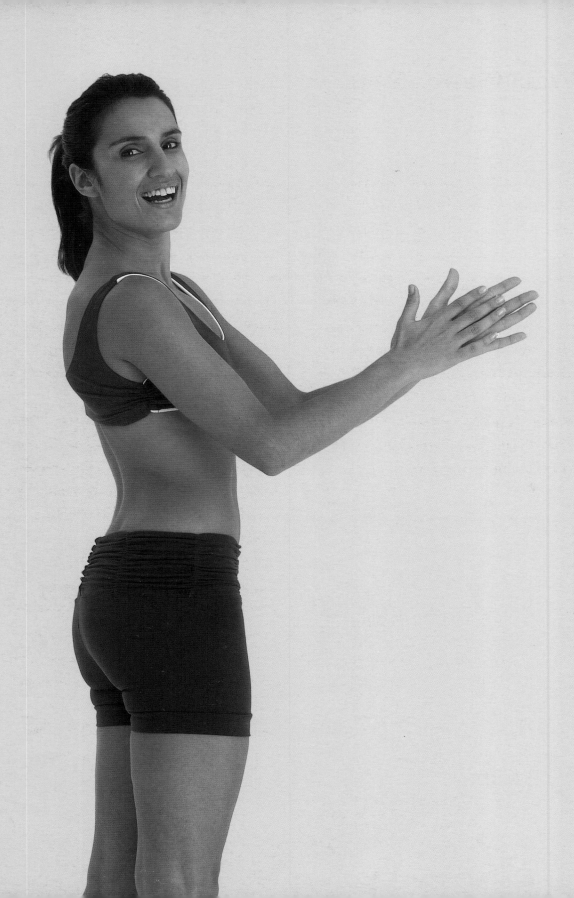

Four Weeks Plus

Congratulations! You have completed the four-week programme and are now hopefully enjoying your new shape and your new flexibility and strength. Having seen the amazing results you can achieve with Pilates, we hope you will want to continue with your training. However, we would recommend that you lighten your schedule a little. You have been through an intensive body-conditioning programme in order to get maximum results in a short period of time and it would be counter-productive to continue at this pace.

We suggest you reduce your training to two or three hours a week. Try to vary your workouts by adding exercises from the other body-shape programmes in this book. We also strongly recommend that you try some of our other books and videos (see Further Information overleaf). Start to create your own workouts bearing in mind the advice given on page 8 on how to balance the exercises.

You should maintain your cardiovascular fitness. If you choose to reduce this, do not allow it to fall below the government guidelines of 30 accumulative minutes per day of aerobic activity at least five times a week.

Above all, try to keep your Pilates technique fresh and stimulating by setting yourself new goals. The advanced exercises we included should have given you some idea of just how challenging and exciting Pilates can be. As we said in the opening chapters, in these four weeks you have laid the foundations of your new body. Now it's time to build on these.

Further Information

Other Body Control Pilates books

BODY CONTROL THE PILATES WAY
0 330 36945 8 / £7.99

THE MIND–BODY WORKOUT
0 330 36946 6 / £12.99

PILATES THE WAY FORWARD
0 330 37081 2 / £12.99

THE OFFICIAL BODY CONTROL PILATES MANUAL
0 330 39327 8 / £12.99

PILATES GYM
0 330 48309 9 / £12.99

THE BODY CONTROL PILATES BACK BOOK
0 330 48311 0 / £9.99

THE BODY CONTROL PILATES
POCKET TRAVELLER
0 330 49106 7 / £4.99

INTELLIGENT EXERCISE WITH PILATES & YOGA
0 330 49389 2 / £12.99

THE PERFECT BODY THE PILATES WAY
0 330 48953 4 / £12.99

PILATES PLUS DIET
0 330 48954 2 / £10.99

THE COMPLETE CLASSIC PILATES METHOD
0 330 41237 X / £12.99

These are available from all good bookshops,
or can be ordered direct from:
Book Services By Post
PO Box 29
Douglas
Isle of Man IM99 IBQ
Credit card hotline +44 (0) 1624 675 137
Postage and packing free in the UK

Pilates Classes and Teacher Training

For general information on the Body Control Pilates
Method; to find a qualified teacher; for information on
how to become a teacher; and for details on books, videos
and other products, please visit the Body Control Pilates
website at www.bodycontrol.co.uk
or write to:

The Body Control Pilates Association
6, Langley Street,
London, WC2H 9JA,
England

Four Week Intensive Body Control Pilates programmes are available at:

The Body Control Pilates Studio
David Lloyd Club
Point West
116 Cromwell Road
London SW7 4XR
England
Tel: 0207 2448060

Clothing

All clothing kindly supplied by
CandidaFaria Ltd
27 Gloucester Place
London W1U 8HU
Collections available from www.candidafaria.com
general switchboard 01639 842 482

Useful Addresses

If you live within the M25 in the UK we can
wholeheartedly recommend the Pure Package – a unique
new healthy gourmet-meal home-delivery service.
A simply delicious way to manage your weight.
www.purepackage.com
Tel: 08456 123888

Watch out for new titles!